Wherever You Are

"*Wherever You Are* answers the question 'What makes a life worth living?' […] A beautifully written love story by a courageous woman who finds the capacity to experience joy and love in the face of devastating loss."
—Maureen Murdock, author of *Unreliable Truth: On Memoir and Memory*

"…a heartwarming reminder of love, commitment, marriage and how to make your way forward after the unimaginable. Lim's honest prose and compelling story… is a wonderful account of all of the emotions, heartbreak, acceptance and ultimately small joys that come with a 'slowed down life.' As life moves forward for all of us, the lesson is to continually accept the new shape of our lives.
—Lee Woodruff, author of In An Instant: A Family's Journey of Love and Healing

"I can't get this story out of my head. It haunts me. It makes me wonder, Would I be that brave? That strong? That full of joy?"
—Jennie Nash, Founder and Chief Creative Officer, AuthorAccelerator.com

"If you're a caregiver for someone who has life changing health issues, or know a caregiver, grab this book. With depth and brutal honesty, Cynthia Lim shares her journey and hard-won lessons about life after her husband's heart attack and resulting brain injury. In this beautifully written memoir she learns gratitude…. Ultimately this is a love story; a marriage and a family that has held fast in spite of overwhelming challenges.
—Barbara Abercrombie, author of A *Year of Writing Dangerously* and *Kicking in the Wall*

Wherever You Are

A Memoir of Love, Marriage, and Brain Injury

Cynthia Lim

To alison,
with appreciation,
Cynthia

cp

coffeetown**press**

Kenmore, WA

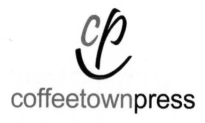

coffeetownpress

For more information go to: www.coffeetownpress.com
www.cynthialimwriting.com

This is a work of nonfiction. Real names have been used with permission; others have been changed.

Cover design by Sabrina Sun
Author photo by GoldWongPhotography

Wherever You Are
Copyright © 2018 by Cynthia Lim

ISBN: 978-1-60381-721-9 (Trade Paper)
ISBN: 978-1-60381-722-6 (eBook)

Library of Congress Control Number: 2018947673

Printed in the United States of America

ACKNOWLEDGEMENTS

I am grateful for everyone who has helped me develop as a writer and for getting this story to publication.

Various chapters of this book were previously published as essays (in a revised form). Chapter 13 was published as "My Absolution" *Gemini Magazine*, Chapter 17 was published as "A Life Worth Living" in *Hawai'i Pacific Review*, Chapter 19 was published as "Rezo para Obtener Favores (I Pray for Blessings)" in *Rougarou: an Online Literary Journal*, Chapter 21 was published as "Yes or No" in *The Legendary*, Chapter 27 was published as "A World of Pain" in *Forge Journal*, Chapter 36 was published as "Flytime" in *Wild Violet Literary Magazine*, Chapter 37 was published as "The Gum Chewing Notary" in *Kaleidoscope: Exploring the Experience of Disability Through Literature and the Fine Arts*, and Chapter 38 was published as "Night Terrors" in *Hobart*. I thank the editors of these fine publications for publishing early pieces of this work.

To my agent, Paul S. Levine, thank you for your persistence and not giving up on me. Thank you to Catherine Treadgold, Jennifer McCord and Aubrey Anderson at Coffeetown Press for their belief in me as a first-time author.

Thank you to Sharon Bray, my first instructor at the UCLA Extension Writer's Program, who helped open the path to writing. Thank you to Barbara Abercrombie for continued guidance and gentle but critical feedback. I benefited from so many of her writer's retreats and literary salons, sharing my work with gifted writers. Thank you to Jennie Nash, book coach extraordinaire, for helping to shape this book and holding my hand through the publication process.

I owe a heap of gratitude to my "Venice Grind" writer's group, Loren Stephens, Yasmin Tong and Robert Goldman for helping me craft this story. This book would not have been possible without your feedback from our monthly workshops and the encouragement to keep writing. Thank you to Deidre Harris for joining our group and helping us maintain the impetus to write.

I am grateful for all the people who have supported us on this journey. I am thankful for the Acquired Brain Injury Program at Santa Monica College for the wide range of programs and resources they offer and the loving support from Jami Evans. Thank you to Geri Knorr for her continued support. I am thankful to the entire staff of the Office of Data and Accountability at the Los Angeles Unified School District who provided me sustenance and reinforcement during tough times as their leader and especially to Yolanda Pompey, Grace Pang Bovy and John Pirone for their daily care and support. I thank Richard Havel for his guidance through financial and legal issues and always lending a helping hand. Thank you to Orly and Ed Burg, who are always there for us.

I am especially thankful for "family who are friends and friends who are family," as quoted by my dear friend Nancy Schmidt. Without the daily support from Nancy and Manny Castellanos, I would be lost. Thank you for the Friday night martinis, late night whiskeys and heartfelt conversations. Thank you to Anthony, Jamie and David Castellanos for being part of the family.

Our siblings and their families have been a great source

of comfort and support: Donna and Philip Yan, Gregory Lim, Jeanne and Kinzen Wong, the late Rosemary Davis and her husband, Ernie Davis, Susan Foreman, and Amy and Tyler Goulston. I thank my niece, Kellie Davis, for her kind and caring visits. A special thank you to my aunt, Georgina Hum and her husband, David Sheridan, for being with me during the darkest hours and celebrating with me during shining moments.

Thank you to Arnold Batongbakal whose competent and devoted caregiving made my life possible. Most of all, thank you to my sons, Zachary and Paul Landsberg, for their strength and fortitude on this journey. I am so proud of the men they have become and continue to be amazed by their kindness and sensitivity. At the heart of this story is Perry, the love of my life, and I am thankful that he was there to receive and express it.

CHAPTER 1

—☀—

I should have started CPR, but when I heard my husband gasp, when I saw his chest heave, I didn't know what to do. Panic rose in my throat like bile.

"Perry!" No response. I shook his shoulder. "Perry!"

Was he breathing? I reached across him to pick up the phone next to the bed and dialed 911. I got the hotel operator.

"Help me, my husband isn't breathing!"

The line disconnected. I jabbed at the buttons, frantic. Another phone rang but it was in the sitting area, twenty feet away. I scrambled off the bed and grabbed the phone. It was the 911 operator.

"Do you know CPR?"

"Yes, I think so," I said, "I don't know. I took it ten years ago. I don't remember. What do I do, what do I do?" I heard my voice rising.

"Stay calm," she said. "Remove any pillows from behind his head."

I dropped the phone and ran back to the bed, pulled the pillows from behind Perry's head and tossed them to the floor. His eyes were still closed and he was not moving. I ran back to the phone.

"Is he breathing?" she asked. "Can you move him to the floor so he can lay flat?"

There was a knock at the door. A man from the front desk appeared, an apparition in white with shoulder length blonde, wispy hair, so pale his eyebrows looked transparent.

"What can I do to help?" he asked in soft voice.

The 911 lady had mentioned CPR, but I couldn't form the words to say it to the blonde man. "Help me move him to the floor," I said as we both started toward the bed.

He reached under Perry's shoulders while I lifted his legs as we transferred him to the floor. I ran back to the phone.

"The paramedics are on their way," the operator said. "I am going to stay on the line with you until they arrive."

I listened to her voice while I looked at Perry, who was lying on the floor with his eyes closed. The man from the hotel stood by watching, too. Was Perry turning blue? You hear people use the phrase 'paralyzed with fear,' but before that moment, I hadn't understood what it meant. I couldn't move. I couldn't act. I stood, listening to the voice of the 911 operator, knowing that there was probably something else I should have been doing, but unable to move.

Then I heard sirens and in minutes, paramedics swarmed the room, two of them, then four, then six, carrying oxygen tanks and what looked like giant toolboxes.

"You may want to step outside, ma'am," said one of the paramedics, taking the phone from my hand.

But I still couldn't move. My feet were rooted to the floor and my eyes were locked on Perry's body.

IT WAS SUPPOSED TO HAVE been a quick overnight trip to Portland, Oregon that weekend of June 6, 2003. Fly up on Friday for the family bar mitzvah on Saturday, then fly back to Los Angeles—twenty-four hours carved out of a hectic home and work life. Perry, a bankruptcy attorney, was nearing the peak of his career at age forty-seven. He was due to leave on a business trip the following week. I worked as an administrator for the Los Angeles Unified School District and had just returned from a conference on data analysis the day before.

Perry and I juggled home and work responsibilities, although our two sons were nearing the age where they didn't need much attention from us. Zack, our older son at eighteen, had just graduated from high school and was starting college in the fall. Paul was fifteen and finishing his freshman year in high school.

The bar mitzvah was for the son of Perry's cousin, Laurie, and her husband Gary, both rabbis. I had asked Perry if it was worth it, this quick trip on an already busy weekend. We were scheduled to attend a reunion at Zack's elementary school on Sunday in Los Angeles.

"Family is important," Perry said. "We should make the effort. Plus my Aunt Isa and cousin Marc are coming all the way from Florida."

Things got complicated after we booked our flights. Zack and Paul's roller hockey team won a qualifying game for the championship, which would be played on the Friday night we were supposed to leave. Perry rescheduled flights so that the two of us would fly to Portland first, then the boys would come after their hockey game that night. The timetable was carefully orchestrated: one of the hockey moms would take them to the airport after the game to catch a flight to San Francisco, then they'd switch planes to Portland.

That Friday afternoon, when Perry and I flew to Portland together, we savored the hours we had together without the boys. Even though we had been married over twenty years, moments alone together were rare. We checked into the hotel, then explored the downtown neighborhood. In the evening, we had dinner with his cousin Marc. All through dinner, we had been tethered to the boys via cell phone. First, the jubilant call, "We won! We're the champions!" Then calls from the airport, "We made it to the gate," "We landed in San Francisco and are boarding for Portland now."

After dinner, Perry and I strolled to Powell's bookstore and by 11:00 p.m. we were in our hotel room waiting for midnight when we would leave to pick up the boys from the airport. Perry dozed on the bed at the Benson Hotel, while I read a book—*Sixpence House*, by Paul Collins, which I had just bought at Powell's. I checked my watch. One more hour to go. Then I heard Perry gasp, saw his chest heave with a sharp intake of breath.

THE PARAMEDICS BEGAN CPR BUT Perry was still, silent, not breathing. After a dozen compressions, they seemed to have given up. One of them unpacked the defibrillator. Were they moving in slow motion? Or was it that they could not move as fast as my heart was beating? It seemed like hours passed before paddles were placed on Perry's chest to administer shocks. Once. Twice.

"A heartbeat!" said one of the paramedics. "We need to intubate!"

I couldn't watch but I couldn't move.

"He's aspirating!" I heard one of the paramedics say as Perry coughed.

A flurry of activity surrounded him, blocking his body from my view. He was loaded onto a gurney and moved out to the hallway.

"You can ride in the front with me," said one of the paramedics, guiding me toward the door. Her blonde hair was pulled back into a ponytail and she was slim, like a model. I looked at the floor littered with wrappings from bandages, syringes and other medical detritus. There was a bright orange stain on the carpet where Perry had aspirated. *Was it the cioppino he had for dinner?* I stopped. What did I need to take with me? My shoes. All I brought to Portland were sandals and dress shoes. My journal. My cell phone charger. His wallet. *My toes will get cold. I need socks. I only have my thin sweater. I need to reach the boys.* I grabbed Perry's dress socks and stuffed them in my tote bag. When I reached the open doorway, a woman from the hotel stopped me.

"Is there anything I can do?" she asked. I stared at her for a few seconds, bewildered. What needed to be done other than get him to the hospital?

"I need to reach my sons," I blurted. "They are landing at midnight and they are expecting us to pick them up."

I jotted down their cell phone number and rushed out the door to the service elevator where the paramedics were waiting.

"We're going to Oregon Health Sciences University Hospital," the ambulance driver said, as I slid into the front seat. "They have the best cardiac care in the state of Oregon."

As we raced off, sirens blaring, I heard voices from the back calling to Perry.

"Oh, maybe he is conscious," said the ambulance driver. "It's a good sign that they are calling his name."

Instead of heading toward the lights of downtown, we climbed up a forested hill, into blackness. The heavy ambulance swerved and swayed around hairpin turns until we reached the emergency entrance of the hospital. I jumped out of the front seat, but before I could turn around to see where the gurney was going, a woman ushered me to a private room. I have no recollection of what she looked like or what she said but I must have given her the basic facts, his name, date of birth, insurance coverage. I didn't remember telling her that he had complained of indigestion after dinner and that we'd stopped and bought him Rolaids after we went to Powell's, or that he was being treated by our family doctor for heartburn and she gave him a prescription for acid reflux, or that he was on Lipitor but had lost a lot of weight in the last two years and his cholesterol was down to normal. All of those facts were noted on his intake form so it must have come from me. I only remembered that she gave me a consent form to sign, and then left the room.

A few minutes later, another woman came into the room.

"Is there anything I can do for you?" she asked. "I'm the

hospital social worker."

They were being so nice to me—a private room, personal service. I didn't know how to answer. Was he alive? Was he going to be able to walk out of this hospital?

I shook my head and she left. There were four or five hard-backed plastic chairs in the room along with a coffee table with magazines and bright fluorescent lights. I sat in one of the chairs and swung my legs, not knowing what to do with my hands. I reached for my cell phone and called Zack, hitting the "Call" button over and over even though I knew they were still in the air, they could not have landed yet. It went to voicemail immediately.

I fished out my journal and jotted, "If there is a God, he would help me now."

I prayed: "Please God, don't let him slip away. He's too young to take leave of this world."

Over and over, I told myself, "He will survive, he must survive."

WAS IT ONLY A FEW hours ago when I looked in the mirror at the Benson Hotel and thought, "*What a wonderful life we have?*" We had worked so hard to get to this place in life—successful in our careers, our kids in private schools and fortunate to have the financial means to take a quick weekend jaunt to Portland. It didn't seem that long ago that we were VISTA volunteers living off subsistence wages and pooling our food stamp allotment. Earlier that day at the airport, Perry had upgraded our seats to first class using his frequent flier miles.

"Why are you wasting your miles on this trip?" I asked. "Save them for a longer trip, when we take our next family vacation."

But he smiled, then planted a kiss on my lips. "What better time than now? Let's indulge, it's just you and me."

We sipped cocktails in the Red Carpet lounge, then lunched on raw vegetable salads during the flight. It had seemed so excessive, all this luxury for such a short flight. When we were approaching the landing in Portland, I reached for his hand like I always did, because flying made me nervous. When the wheels hit the tarmac with a bump and screech, I tightened my grasp. Perry flexed his muscles, his show of strength as my protector.

IN THE HOSPITAL WAITING ROOM, I didn't scream, although every cell in my body was telling me I should. Cold seeped through the linoleum floor. I put on Perry's socks. My back ached from the stiff chair. I found an outlet and plugged my cell phone into the charger. When the doctor from the emergency room opened the door, it felt as if I had been there for an hour but it had only been twenty minutes.

"The paramedics saved your husband's life," he said. "He had a massive cardiac arrest but he's stabilized. The cardiologist is seeing him now."

Relief filled my body. Perry was alive. I called Zack's phone again and again and got voicemail. On my 15th or 20th try, I reached him.

"What's going on? I have about 30 missed calls," he said.

"It's your dad," I said, panic creeping into my voice. "He's had a massive heart attack. I don't know what's going on. You have to come to the hospital. Take a cab from the airport."

My hand was shaking as I read the address of the hospital from the intake form but I couldn't seem to stop it. Then the cardiologist appeared and led me through the corridor to Perry's room. Outside the doorway, he stopped.

"Your husband suffered two insults to his body," he said, in a clipped British accent. I focused on the gap between his two upper front teeth. "The first insult was a massive heart attack due to an irregular heart beat and a clogged artery. The second insult was to his brain. Because his heart stopped, he stopped breathing. Because no resuscitation was initiated, and I'm not blaming you for not performing CPR," he added, touching my arm, "your husband had no oxygen flowing to his brain and may have suffered brain damage. Between the time he stopped breathing and the arrival of the paramedics, he was without oxygen for five to seven minutes. Anything longer than four minutes has severe consequences for brain damage."

My mind tried to process this information. Heart attack? Five to seven minutes? Brain damage? But he's only forty-seven. We just came to Portland for 24 hours. He has a business trip coming up. We have vacation plans. The doctor's words— *"Because no resuscitation was initiated, and I'm not blaming you for not performing CPR"*—pinged somewhere deep inside me, but not in a place I would be able to hear for many years to come.

"Our immediate action is to perform an angioplasty to open up the artery with a stent," he continued. "As with any procedure, I have to inform you of the risks."

He looked into my eyes. I nodded but the words weren't really sinking in. I was floating away, this wasn't my life.

"The risks are severe bleeding, or stroke, in rare cases. But I've already performed six today." He handed me a consent form on a clipboard. "The risk of not doing it at all is, of course, death."

The boys arrived at that moment, ushered in by an emergency room nurse. Zack came through the door first, alarm and seriousness on his face. He inherited my Chinese features and my straight black hair, which was now flattened under the baseball cap emblazoned with "Champions 2003" stitched across a pair of hockey sticks. Paul trailed behind and greeted me with a smile that turned to a frown when he registered the shock on my face. At fifteen, he was nearly as tall as his six foot brother, but his thin brown hair and fair skin resembled Perry's. I hugged them one at a time, relieved that I was no longer alone.

Once I gave my consent, the nursing staff wheeled Perry into the operating room and suddenly the fear and panic that I had been holding in was unleashed. I dissolved into sobs and clung to the boys. We finally retreated to separate chairs, exhausted and spent, and waited.

After a long two hours, the cardiologist appeared. "He was given sedatives but he should wake after 24 hours," the doctor said. "If he doesn't wake within 48 hours, the consequences are dire. The survival rate is not high; there is only a 50% chance of survival. Of those that do survive, they suffer some form of permanent disability. Full recovery is rare." He paused, letting us take in the news. "He is being taken back to intensive care and you will be able to see him shortly. Do you have a place to stay?" he asked. "You may be in town for awhile."

IT WAS FIVE IN THE morning when I finally climbed into bed at the hotel but I couldn't sleep. What if Perry died? What would I be without Perry? Even after twenty years of marriage, I still felt the same bone-tingling excitement when his eyes lit up and he smiled at me. We could be surrounded by noise and kids and family but he could always make me feel as if I was the only person in the room.

"I hope I die before you do because I cannot picture life without you," I had said to him once.

He laughed and said, "Cyn, you know that's not how it's going to happen. Women outlive men. I'll be long gone before you."

My heart had tightened with fear at the thought. I could not imagine a life without him. But now there was another fear. What if he was brain damaged? What would he be like without a fully functioning brain? What would become of our marriage, our home, our family, our life? And somewhere at the edges of everything, still too deep to be a conscious thought, was the tiny ping, the little alarm: Was I to blame?

CHAPTER 2

–⁄‹–

Perry and I met the first day of college at UC Santa Barbara.
"Is this the line to register your bike?" asked a nasally
voice behind me.

I turned and there was Perry, his wispy brown hair almost
touching his shoulders, a gold stud in his right ear, and a broad
smile revealing even white teeth. Under his faded denim
overalls, he wore a purple tee shirt with a grinning Cheshire
Cat, and no shoes. I was intrigued by his appearance. In
1974, there were not many men in my hometown of Salinas,
California who sported earrings.

"Where are you from?" he asked.

"Salinas," I said. "It's inland from Monterey."

"I'm from Torrance," he said. "Do you know where that is?
Near L.A.?"

I shook my head. I had only been to Los Angeles twice in
my life, both times to visit Disneyland.

"I drive through Salinas all the time when I go backpacking
in Big Sur," he said. "Do you backpack?"

"No," I said. My only experience camping was a night
spent at a drive-in campground with my Girl Scout troop in

the fourth grade. I woke to find a pincher bug in my shoe. When I got home, my mother scrubbed me head to toe. As an immigrant from China, the idea of camping out was foreign to her. "Camping is so dirty," she said, "Why would you want to go sleep out in the dirt when you have a nice, clean house with comfortable beds?"

"You remind me of someone I know," Perry said. "She has hair like yours." I was flattered that he noticed my waist-length black hair. That morning, I had used my electric curlers on the ends to give it more bounce. I was wearing my favorite light blue gauze top embroidered with lavender and green flowers, my faded bell bottom jeans, and brown sandals with one-inch cork heels, which put me eye-to-eye with Perry. When he lifted his hand to push away a lock of hair, I saw a black bracelet tied in a knot around his wrist.

"It's an elephant hair bracelet that a friend of mine gave me," he said, holding out his arm. "She's from Africa."

Everything about him seemed unusual, even his name. As we progressed through the line, I learned that he just liked to talk and he filled any pause in the conversation with jokes. *"Did you hear the one about the three bad eggs? Two bad."* By the time our bicycles were registered, I knew that he had split with his high school girlfriend because she was going to Berkeley and he didn't believe in long distance relationships; that he had worked at a record store and bought himself a new stereo system for his dorm room; that his job before that was at the Gap, where he bought his college wardrobe; that his family was Jewish but they didn't go to temple; and that his mother loved to cook so I should come to his house for dinner sometime in Torrance. He invited me to his dorm room that night because he'd brought a huge chunk of hash in case he couldn't find drugs in Santa Barbara. We smoked that soap-sized chunk of hash all through our first quarter in college.

THERE WAS NO ROMANCE BETWEEN us for the first six months. He was pursuing several women in his dorm and I got involved with a junior who lived off campus in Isla Vista. As we studied in Perry's dorm room or ate in the dining commons, I learned that he felt out of place being Jewish in lily-white Torrance. I felt the same being Chinese in Salinas. Perry seemed worldly compared to my sheltered upbringing. He had attended concerts at the Roxy and Troubadour on the Sunset Strip, while the only concerts I went to were at the Monterey County Fairgrounds. In high school, he frequented art exhibits at museums and galleries, while in Salinas my friends and I cruised Main Street or drove out to country roads among the lettuce fields for fun. He teased me about being a country bumpkin, as if I had lived in a cave for seventeen years. It wasn't far from the truth.

When we came back to school after that first Christmas break, Perry was really happy to see me.

"I've been thinking about us a lot over vacation," he said. I'd never seen him so serious. "I think we should be more than just friends."

He grabbed my hand to draw me close, but I wasn't ready. I liked being friends. I liked our easy banter without the tension of romance. I twisted my hands free and escaped to the other side of his dorm room, then sank into his bean bag chair.

"I don't know," I said. "Let me think about it."

What about all the women he was always telling me about? Perry was goofy, he was my best friend, my buddy, not someone I would fall in love with and swoon over. Besides, my Grandma, whom I loved more than anyone in the world, wanted me to marry someone Chinese.

Perry was patient but persistent. He appeared at my dorm every night, sought me out in the dining hall, made plans to see me every weekend. By February, I was looking forward to seeing him, too. It seemed to happen overnight when I looked at him with different eyes; suddenly he was someone I wanted to spend all of my time with. I can't even remember what tugged at my heart—the intensity in his eyes when he looked at me or his mouth that always curved into a smile that made me giggle. After we became lovers, each touch triggered bone-tingling excitement. The other women, the other men, fell away. We became inseparable and absorbed in each other. As the school year drew to a close, we despaired about the coming summer. I had to return to Salinas to work at the family grocery store. Perry was staying in Santa Barbara and we counted out the weeks that we would be apart, vowing to write to each other every day, and to never spend another summer apart.

In those twenty-eight years since our freshman year in college, we had only spent a handful of nights away from each other. When he traveled on business he would fly at impossible times in the dead of night to get home as quickly as possible. That night in Portland, as I lay in bed listening to Zack and Paul's soft breathing, I felt as if I had stepped onto a foreign planet without Perry at my side.

CHAPTER 3

—◦—

At seven the next morning, I woke with a start. What was it the cardiologist said? Perry had to wake up in the next 24 hours. The clock was ticking. I roused the boys to return to the hospital. We stopped in the hospital cafeteria so the boys could eat—they were always hungry. But I was still in shock as I sat at a table with my hands wrapped around a cup of hot chocolate, trying to warm the chill in my body. I shivered in my thin sweater and sandals, even though I had put on Perry's socks.

In the intensive care unit, Perry was hooked to monitors and machines. I squeezed his hand, hoping that the strength of my touch would bring him back.

"Fight Perry, fight," I whispered in his ears. "Wake up in the next 24 hours."

Cousin Marc drifted in. There was a call from Aunt Isa. Various nurses and doctors did their rounds. I stationed myself at Perry's side, clutching his hand, listening to the rhythmic gasping and sighing of the respirator and the beeping of the heart monitor. I thought I felt his hand tighten and grasp mine in return but the nurse shook her head.

"Posturing," she said. "It's a sign of brain damage."

There wasn't much we could do for Perry, but there were a thousand mundane details that needed attention: calls to Perry's sister in Sacramento, my aunt, my siblings, our neighbors, the friends who were expecting to see us at the school reunion on Sunday. There were our flights, the rental car, the dog in a kennel and the fact that we had only packed enough clothes for one day.

Zack sprang into action. "Why don't I fly home with Paul, take care of the dog, get us some more clothes and other stuff we need?" he said. "I can make all the calls to the law firm and your work. I think it's going to be a long haul."

I wondered what would happen with Perry's work, my work. He had taken the LSAT on a lark after undergraduate school and received high scores. His decision to go to law school seemed so casual, flippant almost. But then he did well in law school, got recruited by a big law firm in Los Angeles and made partner a year early. His financial success had allowed me to stay home with the boys for five years, then go back to school for a doctorate. I had only been back at work full time for three years, but I had a career that was fulfilling and stimulating. In two weeks, I was scheduled to attend a conference in Washington D.C. What would happen to me now?

THE NEXT DAY, ZACK AND Paul flew home and Amy, Perry's sister, arrived from Sacramento. The days melted together in a swirl of tests and doctors. In this teaching hospital, there was a new face every day and I lost track of who was who. Amy and I finally met with all the doctors in one room: the cardiologist, two residents, an intern, the senior doctor, the neurologist. Up until then, my faith in doctors had been complete, trusting. My contact with doctors had always been for happy occasions, like the birth of our sons. They were infallible in my eyes. Now, each one offered differing opinions. One had said the prognosis was grim if he didn't wake up in 48 hours. Another mentioned 24. Was it 24 or 48 hours? And what did a grim prognosis mean anyway?

"When patients wake after 24 hours or less, there is little resultant brain damage. Prognosis for recovery is very good," said the neurologist. "However, after 72 hours or more, chances for full recovery decrease. The longer the coma, the greater the extent of brain damage. We won't know the extent of brain damage until he wakes from his coma. If he wakes from his coma."

If? I looked back at their faces. *No, not Perry. He's going to wake from this coma, he's a fighter.* They didn't know how smart Perry was, how persistent. He was going to wake up. He had to.

"But what does this mean?" I asked, scanning their faces. "What is the best case? What is the worst case?"

The senior doctor glanced at his colleagues, then stepped forward and cleared his throat. I concentrated on his face, his full head of gray hair, mussed up as if he had just woken up, and his crooked bottom teeth.

"He hasn't regained consciousness and it's been over 48 hours. It could be a sign that he is shutting down and will expire in a week or so. That's the worst case scenario."

Expire? No! That's not going to happen. He wouldn't leave me in this way. I took a deep breath but it seemed as if all the air had already been sucked out of the room.

"Or he can remain in a coma indefinitely, possibly in a vegetative state, and we would have to make some judgment about life support and end of life decisions," he said, in a low, soft voice.

I imagined Perry forever in this state, lying in a bed with a breathing tube, hooked to monitors in an institution somewhere. *Oh God, what if he never wakes up? What if he remains a vegetable for the rest of his life?*

"The best case scenario is that he wakes immediately. Even though he's been in a coma for more than 48 hours, he could recover from this completely, but it would take months of recovery and rehabilitation before he could conceivably go back to work. Brain injury is individualized, there's no typical case, no typical course of recovery. So even if he woke today, you are looking at months of rehabilitation and a strong likelihood of permanent disability."

After the conference, Amy and I walked outside the building to the gazebo at the top of Marquam Hill. I took several deep breaths but couldn't seem to get enough oxygen in my lungs. *Permanent disability.* It was the first time that word entered my consciousness. Stretched out below was a stunning view of Portland and the Willamette River but all I could see were the wisps of my dreams and future plans, dissipating in the cloudy skies.

I remembered my mother's reaction when my father and grandfather were killed in a plane crash when I was seven. She took to her bed for days, then weeks, leaving her five children, my maternal grandmother and my ten-year-old aunt to grieve on our own. She emerged with eyes red and swollen, helpless and vulnerable. An immigrant from China with limited English, she was dependent on my father's business partners to help her with the grocery business. But they never treated her as an equal partner. She had no say in business decisions and was never kept aware of how much money the business was making. Her income and work hours were dictated by the partners and her expenses closely scrutinized. I saw how her personality was shaped from that day forward: tentative, insecure, suspicious of others. She relied on her children for translation, driving and navigating the English-speaking world. I had hated that feeling of dependency, of my mother depending on us children and depending on her business partners, all because we no longer had a father.

"I am going to be just like my mother," I said to Amy as I sobbed, imagining how our lives would change.

"No, you are not," said Amy, wrapping me in a hug. "You will get through this. You are not your mother!"

As I wiped the tears from my face, I knew I had to stay strong. I had to put up a brave front for Zack and Paul to give them assurance that we would be okay, even if I didn't know what would happen. As a child, I had vowed that I would never be in the same predicament as my mother. I would not wallow in self-pity. I would understand and direct my own finances. I would not depend on anyone for my livelihood or my happiness or my well-being. But I realized that now, it was going to take every ounce of strength I could summon.

CHAPTER 4

～✶～

For the next week, I woke disoriented each morning, not sure of where I was. Then I would remember: I was in Portland, Perry was in a coma, we didn't know if and when he would wake. It seemed impossible that the sun was shining, that the sky was clear blue, and that I could hear birds chirping outside our window. My life had been upended and yet for the rest of the world, normal routines resumed.

How easy it would have been to give in to grief and burrow my head under the covers and never emerge. Visitors had come to offer comfort: Perry's cousins in Portland, two of Perry's partners from his law firm and my aunt Georgina who organized meals, drove me to the hospital and stayed with the boys so that I could be at Perry's side. I so wanted to surrender everything to them and retreat in sorrow.

At the hospital, when Paul collapsed in sobs, heaving uncontrollably, I knew what my mother's helplessness must have felt like. I could offer Paul no words of comfort, no assurances that everything would be okay. All I could do was hold him in my arms and pat his back. I had to be strong. I saw the alarm on Paul's face when I cried, how he would rush to hold my hand or give me a hug whenever tears formed in my eyes.

I tried to suppress the fear growing inside me that nothing would ever be the same again. Rich, Perry's friend from his law firm, flew up for the day and sat at his bedside holding his hand. Over lunch, he explained that the law firm had started the application for disability insurance.

"If he remains disabled, the firm will pay his full income through the end of the year, and then the disability payments should start in January," he said. He slid a manila envelope toward me with a copy of the policy. "It's a generous benefit amount, plus Perry bought supplemental insurance."

I fingered the envelope, absorbing Rich's words. They already knew it was unlikely that Perry would be able to resume his career as an attorney. I felt a lump form in my throat. What would become of us, of our lifestyle? Thank God Perry had always been fiscally conservative. We still lived in our 1,100 square foot "starter home" in Mar Vista while most of his partners had moved to tonier neighborhoods with more rooms and hefty mortgages. We had amassed a nest egg for the boys' college education, for family vacations, and as Perry always said, "In case anything bad happens to us and we need to survive for at least a year." We would probably still be able to afford college and private schools, but a feeling of anxiety washed over me. Would it be enough?

I was grateful that I had my own career and salary, even though it wasn't enough to sustain our current lifestyle. I put the envelope with the disability policy in my purse. *It would have to be enough. I will make it work.* Perry and I had always been equal partners when it came to finances. After college, we combined our meager resources. As our income grew, we still shared everything and never questioned each other's expenditures. At least I knew all the details of our financial state.

By the time Zack and Paul returned to Portland with suitcases loaded with our clothes, books, and mail, I had moved us to a two-bedroom suite at the Residence Inn with a full kitchen. Zack was stoic and immersed himself in writing a blog to inform family and friends on Perry's progress. In 2003, blogs were not common vocabulary then, but Zack researched how to create a live journal. Paul shrank into the background, morose and glum. I could see the sorrow in his eyes when he held Perry's hand. They were fishing buddies; they traveled all over the state and to Mexico on fishing excursions. At least once a month, they rose early on Saturday mornings and went out on Perry's fishing boat to Malibu or Palos Verdes.

Perry had signed Paul up for a wilderness course in Wyoming that was starting the following week. I remembered how they had both been so excited about the trip, poring over the catalogue, discussing the flight schedule. I wondered if it would help, sending Paul on this trip instead of spending hours in the hospital. But what kind of mother let her child go away while their father was in a coma? Besides, what if Perry died while he was gone?

I took a deep breath. No one knew what the outcome for Perry would be. I could put a halt to everyone's lives, mine, Zack's and Paul's like my mother did and insist that we remained huddled next to his bedside. We could live our lives forever in the shadow of his trauma. Or we could carry on. I reached out for Paul's arm.

"If you still want to go on your trip, it's okay with me," I said.

I could see the relief in his eyes. "Dad seems like he is stabilizing and I don't feel like I can do anything for him here," he said.

I hoped that I had made the right decision.

As Paul readied himself for the wilderness trip, the doctors were optimistic that Perry could be transferred home to Los Angeles. But another five days passed with conflicting reports about which hospital would take him and which day he would be transferred. I was torn between staying in Portland to advocate for his transfer or flying home so that I could take Paul to the airport for his wilderness trip. I chose to fly home with Zack so we could be with Paul.

I expected to feel relieved when I got home but I didn't realize how painful it was to be in our house without Perry. When I opened the refrigerator, I saw the new red potatoes that he had bought at Farmer's Market the weekend before we left for Portland. The cupboards held his favorite cheese pretzels and the non-fat Caesar salad dressing he special-ordered after he joined Weight Watchers.

I sat at my computer and read about anoxic encephalopathy, Perry's formal diagnosis. The nurse in Portland had given me handouts when I was in the intensive care unit but it had looked like Sanskrit to me. Now that I was home, I was able to read coherently. Links to medical reports appeared, each more sobering than the first. Chances for recovery were minimal, most people who lost oxygen and survived were faced with significant disabilities for the rest of their lives. I was staring at my fate on the computer screen in stark black and white, but I was in denial. *My life would not come to that,* I thought. I didn't want to believe those dire accounts.

I logged off the computer and picked up an envelope on the desk with Perry and Paul's airline tickets to Mulege, Baja California. They were supposed to leave on a fishing trip in a few weeks. Attached to the ticket was my affidavit affirming that Perry had permission to travel with Paul out of the country. Just a month earlier, Perry and I had raced around town on a Saturday to get the affidavit notarized. I was annoyed at having to take time out of my precious weekend and we argued in the car. Now, I felt regret for ever being angry at him or having cross words with him. The thought he may not even survive the coma loomed in the back of my mind.

My feelings of helplessness and surrender returned. How was I ever going to have the strength to continue on like this? I fought the impulse to climb into bed, inhale Perry's scent on the pillow and weep. But Zack and Paul were urging me to go across the street where my neighbors, Manny and Nancy, were waiting with glasses of cognac. I knew that they were worried sick about us. For the last fifteen years, we had been constant companions and our sons were close in age to their two sons, Anthony and David. We shared weekly dinners, celebrated promotions, birthdays, anniversaries and journeyed into the wilderness together each summer.

That evening, I poured out my fears about Perry's prognosis, the uncertainty of his coma and his return to Los Angeles.

"I may have to fly back to Portland if they can't find a hospital bed for him in Los Angeles," I said.

Manny jumped up.

"Davey plays soccer with a kid whose dad is the head of a hospital in Santa Monica. Let's give him a call."

In a matter of minutes, Manny was on the phone with him, and the next morning at 8 a.m., I received a call from the hospital.

"We have a bed for your husband," said the woman from admissions. "We are calling the hospital in Oregon and your health insurance now to make the arrangements. We could probably get him transferred here by tomorrow."

I was glad that I had chosen to go across the street to Manny and Nancy's rather than go to bed and cry into my pillow. It was a lesson that I would learn over and over in the years to come. I could not do this all on my own. I had to reach out beyond my own grief and learn to embrace the support of others.

CHAPTER 5

꠸꠸꠸

When Perry was finally transferred to a hospital in Santa Monica, the nurse with the Medi-vac team had told us he was waking up. But when Zack and I saw him, it seemed that nothing had changed. We couldn't rouse him and he was still in a coma.

On his second morning in California, however, our family doctor and a nurse were standing next to Perry's bed, laughing and grinning. Perry was on his back with his eyes opened, the sheet pulled off of him.

"He's obeying commands!" the doctor said. "Watch this! Perry, wiggle your right toe." His right toe moved. "Close your left eye." His left eyelid closed. "He is out of his coma!" said the doctor.

I ran to Perry's side and his eyes were open, seeing, following. He saw me and smiled. My heart lurched, my breath caught in my throat.

"Perry!" I cried. He was awake! He pursed his lips to kiss me. My heart melted. He's alive! He's awake! "I love you! I miss you!" I exclaimed. "I'm so happy to see you!"

Perry kept smiling. He squeezed my hand. I rushed outside

to call Zack, then the Outdoor Leadership School to get a message to Paul in Wyoming. When I ran back into the room, Perry's eyes followed me and there was his magnificent smile when I stood next to him. When Zack arrived twenty minutes later, Perry was still awake. His eyes lit up at the sight of Zack's thick black hair and the traces of stubble on his adolescent face.

"Hey Dad!" Zack exclaimed. "What's up?"

Perry moved his mouth as if to talk to us but no words came out. The tracheotomy tube blocked any sound from his vocal cords. We rejoiced over his awakening but after another five minutes of smiling and grinning at us, he fell into a deep sleep again.

I wanted to shout from the rooftops, "He's awake! He's come back!"

MY JOY AND HOPE WERE short-lived. Perry had woken up, but his speech was garbled and nonsensical, and it was never certain whether he understood what we were saying. I feared that he would drift into the recesses of coma again unless I was there to keep his mind occupied and stimulated. Each morning, for the next month, I rushed to the hospital so I could be there when the respiratory therapist infused his tracheotomy tube with mentholated mist to clear his breathing passages. I was there when the speech therapist quizzed him on his vocabulary or fed him Jell-O to work on his swallowing. I hovered nearby when the physical therapist helped him to his feet and let him stand for a few seconds. In the long hours between therapy visits, I read to him and coaxed him to talk.

My strength was flagging. I wondered how long I could sustain this level of effort, how long I could put my own life on hold for Perry's. Since his heart attack, I had completely neglected myself. When I looked in the mirror, I saw dark bags under my eyes and my forehead lined with worry. My short black hair hung flat against my head because I forgot to run a brush through it before I left for the hospital. My complexion was sallow and pale, as if the gray walls of the hospital had leeched the vitality out of me. It was July in Los Angeles and normally, I would be in shorts and tee shirts, my arms and legs brown from the sun. My world now consisted of the metered parking lot near the hospital, the dark cafeteria in the basement with watery coffee and bland casseroles, the antiseptic smell of the hospital ward and the hard plastic chair parked next to Perry's bed. Was this what my life was going to be now?

One day, when Zack came to relieve me at the hospital, he said, "Mom, you need to go back to work. This is not good for you."

I knew he was right. I made arrangements to return to my job.

ON MY FIRST DAY BACK at the office, as I walked past rows of gray clothed cubicles and stained gray and black carpet, I faced rounds of questions from colleagues. How was Perry? How was I? How were the boys? Did I need anything? Could people help? My resolve weakened. Maybe I wasn't doing the right thing, maybe I wasn't strong enough for this yet. But when I reached my desk near the window, at the end of a long row of cubicles, familiarity flooded me. I surveyed my desk and everything was the way I had left it a month ago. Files were still stacked along the credenza, my notebook awaited me. This was evidence that I had another life, another identity other than the wife of a brain-injured patient.

I settled into my chair and swiveled to face the windows. On this clear July morning, I could see a sliver of the ocean, framed by the Baldwin Hills to the south and the Santa Monica mountains to the north. I checked my voicemail messages. I turned on my computer and reacquainted myself with the files spread over my desk, wondering if it would seem like gibberish or if I was even capable of concentrating.

I picked up the draft of a document I had been working on that described data variables and spelled out their values. I remembered this world. Although my formal education was in social work, I had gravitated to research and policy analysis. Now I worked for the school district as an analyst who designed data reports for teachers and administrators. I knew what to do. On my computer, I began typing instructions to programmers on what data tables needed to be built, which table to use to extract a number, what formula to use to derive the measure, how the columns should be labeled, and which variables should be included to disaggregate the measures. My shoulders relaxed as a sense of calm enveloped me. I found comfort in the numbers, fact tables and data structures. This formula, this combination of numbers would always yield the same result and I could count on the sureness of it. Numbers were absolute, certain. This world contained known entities that I could control.

As the days passed, I became absorbed in the data world again. One afternoon, I was startled by the ringing of my cell phone on my desk. It was Paul, wondering what time I would be at the hospital. For those few precious hours in my cubicle, I had forgotten about hospitals, brain injured husbands, unknown recovery paths and unanswered questions. I sighed, then reluctantly rose from my chair. It was time to enter the world of disability again.

CHAPTER 6

~\!/~

In mid-July, Zack and I were standing in his bedroom after another long day at the hospital. "Maybe I should defer college for a year," he said. "I think you need me at home."

"No!" I yelled. The response exploded out of me like a reflex, taking me by surprise. I thought about my mother again, how we became responsible for her happiness after my father died. She made sure her needs came first, above everyone else's. I felt guilty when I went away to college because I was the last child to leave home. Even now, in adulthood, my mother always made us children feel guilty if we neglected her. I did not want to repeat that same pattern with Zack.

I reached for his arm. "No, I will be fine. We will be fine."

I didn't want him to miss out on his college experience. College was all about freedom for me, to pursue my own path, to live my own life. I wanted the same for Zack. I remembered how enthusiastic Perry had been throughout the college application process, how proud he was that Zack had been accepted at NYU, how they visited New York together to tour the campus and art program. Perry had called me from New York to say, "I think it's going to be okay, Cyn. It looks like a city but I always deferred to Perry to plan our itinerary. He was the one that would pick out a restaurant or a play off-Broadway and negotiate taxis and subways. On our last visit several years earlier, we had come without the boys for a long weekend. Perry booked a room at the Plaza, then took me window shopping on Fifth Avenue. We hopped on the subway to Barney Greengrass for whitefish salad, and for dinner, we took a cab to Tribeca. All I had to do was follow along.

But now, as I looked around the cramped hotel room, I wondered if I had the confidence to navigate the city on my own. Outside, I could hear taxis blaring their horns and trucks rumbling down the street. Paul, freshly showered with his hair still wet, emerged from the bathroom and looked at me with raised eyebrows.

"Now what?" he asked.

I took a deep breath. We could just stay inside and wallow in pity in this stuffy hotel room. Or we could go out and explore the city. It was my time to lead, to be the guide. I had to be strong for him and for me.

"Get your shoes on, let's go out."

For the next four hours, Paul and I walked all over the Lower East Side. The forward motion, the sounds of the streets and parade of faces kept my sadness at bay. We wandered past the purple banners hanging from the NYU buildings, through Washington Square and into Greenwich Village for lunch. Then we walked south on Broadway, munching on candied nuts from sidewalk vendors and browsing in bookstores. We kept walking south and ended up in Little Italy at dinner time, charmed by the lights strung across Mulberry Street and the smell of garlic from the restaurants lining the street. We settled into an Italian restaurant and watched the waiter prepare a Caesar salad, Paul's favorite, at our table. I leaned back in my chair, feeling the tiredness in my feet and the stiffness in my neck. I closed my eyes and a sense of satisfaction washed over me. I did it, we came to New York without Perry and we survived.

CHAPTER 7

～、⁄～

I knew that Perry couldn't stay in the hospital forever, but I had no idea what the next step would be or where he would go after the hospital in Santa Monica. When we returned from New York there was a voicemail message that Perry was being moved to a nursing home. I was taken aback—how could this happen without my input?

I had gone down that path before when I was befriended by a woman in the hospital who I assumed was a social worker. She urged me to visit a rehabilitation center for Perry because he needed more stimulation. It turned out to be a nursing home. I remembered the sense of foreboding I felt when I went on a tour and looked at the room they would place him in. Three men were lying silently in their beds, eyes fixed on the television mounted in the corner, their beds parallel to each other. A thin curtain separated each bed and there was barely enough space for a single folding chair between beds. There were no pictures on the end tables, no personal effects to identify their wives, their children, their family or who they used to be. I vowed then that I would never move Perry to a place like that.

He needed to be in a rehabilitation hospital, I was told by the physical and occupational therapists at the hospital. "He needs more aggressive therapy," they told me. But how was I going to make that happen? I knew nothing about rehabilitation or how health insurance worked. What I did know was how to be persistent and pestering. I made dozens of phone calls to our primary care doctor, intake counselors, case managers and anyone I knew in the medical field before I was able to get him transferred to a highly regarded brain rehabilitation center.

I was filled with hope again. How could he not get better if he was placed at the best facility and received the best care? Maybe our lives could return to normal.

I WAS AMAZED BY PERRY'S progress in his first two weeks at the rehabilitation hospital. For the first time since his heart attack, he was upright and could sit at a table and feed himself, his hands shaky as they guided a spoon with pureed food into his mouth. Gone was the hospital gown, replaced by his own shorts, tee shirt and tennis shoes. He brushed his teeth and with the assistance of the attendants, took daily showers. The physical therapist guided him to walk, and by the end of the first week, he was able to walk sixty yards on his own, with a shuffle step and uneven balance. He sat in a wheelchair during the day and learned to propel himself into the corridors of the ward or the community room. His usual cheerful self returned. One day, after walking on his own for a hundred yards, he was jubilant. Zack and Paul stood by, proud and happy.

"Way to go," said Zack, handing him his hat and sunglasses. Perry placed the baseball cap on his head, then slipped on the sunglasses and beamed.

"I'm a stud!" Perry exclaimed.

"You look great, Dad!" said Paul.

"Everyone's been saying that to me," said Perry, in a clear, audible voice. "They keep saying, 'You look good, you look great.'"

For a brief moment, he looked as if there was nothing

wrong with him. He would get better, he would come home. Our former lives seemed within grasp.

I VISITED HIM TWICE EACH day, in the morning before work and late afternoon after work. I usually stayed until he was put to bed in the evening. After the attendant changed him into a hospital gown and pants for the night, I would dim the lights in his room, then chatter about my day, about the boys, about the hospital, about what was troubling me. It was those moments before he went to sleep that I felt he was really present. He would look at me, eyes serious and knowing, seemingly undamaged by brain injury.

On one of those nights, I told him about the strange sound in the tires as I drove the van to work, how I took time off work to go to the tire store but they couldn't find anything wrong and now I had to take more time off so I could get it checked out by a mechanic. He held my face in his hands, his eyes tender and concerned, filled with love.

"Everything falls on you," he said.

I could feel warmth spreading from my heart into my chest and body. He really was coming back.

And then, suddenly, he wasn't.

Toward the end of his second week at the rehabilitation hospital, he was rubbing his front teeth with his index finger one morning, his eyes wide with a faraway look.

"What is it, Perry? Why are you rubbing your teeth?" I asked.

He didn't respond but kept rubbing.

"Does it hurt?" I asked.

He looked at me with distant eyes, not really seeing me. I felt a shiver as goose bumps formed on my arm. What was happening to him? He was in a different world where something in his brain triggered this response and he didn't know how to stop. I reached over, grabbed his hand and held it so he couldn't rub his teeth.

"Is there something wrong with your teeth?" I asked.

"No. I don't know," he replied, looking away, distracted by a group of people walking by. It was the first sign of the agitation in his mind. In the days that followed, he became restless, frustrated from being confined to his wheelchair. I tried to quell my anxiety when the physical therapist and the nurse reported that he kept trying to get out of his wheelchair, even though his balance was off. The attendants tied knots in the seat belt of the wheelchair to prevent him from standing and toppling over. When that failed, they duct taped him into his chair.

One evening, I pulled the tape off and wheeled him out to the patio, then parked his chair near one of the tables. When I looked away, he pushed himself to a couple of tables over, then stood. Before I could get to him, he crumpled to the floor. I ran to him, alarmed.

"I'm okay, I'm okay," he repeated, as I got him back in the chair. "I can stand up."

But he wasn't okay. He wasn't listening to reason and he wasn't aware of his deficits.

As HE BECAME MORE AWAKE and conscious, his brain grew more confused. He would walk into other patient's rooms, holding onto bed frames, tables and the backs of chairs for balance. He tried to open the locked doors on the ward when I wheeled him down the corridors. At random times, he would pull down his pants or peel off his shirt, a crazy, wild-eyed stare in his eyes. I shrank back in panic when he was in this state. I didn't recognize this stranger that inhabited Perry's body and didn't know where this craziness came from.

One night, he insisted that there was a cell phone in his pants and kept trying to pull them off. I got the nurses and attendants to help me get him dressed again. They suggested we go out to the patio. I wheeled him outside and parked next to a table. His brain was still stuck on phones.

"I need to install a phone line," he whispered. "We need two more phone lines for home."

I sat next to him, befuddled. How do I respond to someone who is making no sense? A group of visitors passed our table, on their way into the ward.

"Hey!" Perry hissed. "What's the phone number here?" His voice didn't raise above a whisper and I was relieved that they didn't turn around because they couldn't hear him. He turned to me, desperation in his eyes, "Tell them. Tell them I need a phone!"

The agitation got worse during his third week. Going to the hospital was no longer a joy. I faced each visit with ongoing dread. I never knew what I would find—the compliant Perry or the agitated Perry? One day, as I entered the ward, the nurse saw me and shook her head.

"He's really agitated today. He's been taking off his clothes and getting up from his chair."

I found him in his wheelchair in the hallway, in his tee shirt and hospital pants. I wheeled him back toward his room while he held his arms out to the side to latch on to the wall or door knobs, anything to stop the forward motion. As we passed the doorway to the staff lounge, he hung onto the door knob, wanting to get in.

"No, you can't go in that room," I said to him, reaching around to unclasp his hand from the door knob.

He looked at me with crazed eyes, not recognizing me. As I moved his arm away, he made motions as if he wanted to bite my hand, a fierceness in his eyes that I had never seen before. I pulled my hand back in alarm. He had never been violent with me. Scared, I got the attendants to help. They pushed his wheelchair into his room and changed him into his own shorts. He was in another world, impenetrable and inaccessible to me. He got up from his chair as soon as the attendants left the room, grasped the table, then the chair for balance. He mumbled about phone lines and the need to make a phone call. He walked into the patient's room next door, which was empty, and tried to use the phone. I alerted the nurse who followed him there, coaxing him to return to his own room. She grabbed his arms to guide him, "Come on, Perry. Let's go back to your room. This isn't your room and this isn't your bed."

Perry looked at her with confusion and madness in his eyes. "I need to make a phone call," he insisted.

"Let's go back to your room," the nurse said, holding his arm at the elbow. He swung his arm away to get out of her grasp.

"Call my wife Cynthia," he said, "She helps me."

I stepped forward. "Perry, I'm right here," I said to him. "Here I am."

But he was not seeing me. He was in a world that I could not reach and he was a Perry that I did not recognize. A fear like I had never known rippled through my body. Who was this person that was returning and what would I do with him now?

CHAPTER 8

—✶—

After his fourth week at the rehabilitation hospital, when Perry was at the height of his agitation, I was astounded when they told me he was ready to be discharged. Our insurance had authorized thirty days and they were up. I was in shock and disbelief, wondering how they could possibly consider discharging him now, when he was out of control. What was I supposed to do with him now?

I was terrified of the idea of bringing him home. I couldn't imagine how Zack or Paul or I could handle him in his agitation. Sometimes, it took two attendants and a nurse plus Zack and Paul to get him to stay in his room. What if he woke in the middle of the night and pulled the sheets off the bed? Who would help us if he tried to run out the door or take off all his clothes?

The alternatives were even less appealing—a nursing home or a residential facility, two hours away from Los Angeles. I started to convince myself that once I got him home, he would get better. He would be with me and the boys and our dog Drake, he would get his memory back, he wouldn't be agitated, our lives would return to normal. I repeated this to myself like a mantra, as if believing it would make it come true.

I interviewed a home health care agency and discovered it would cost over $2,300 a week for 24-hour care. I would need almost $10,000 per month. Even with our income from the firm and our little nest egg, our funds would burn through fast at this rate. I found a handy man to install a grab bar in the shower. At a friend's suggestion, I replaced the glass pane in our coffee table with a plastic pane, in case Perry sat on the coffee table.

There was no guidebook to follow and I was grasping for whatever I could find on my own. I scheduled an interview with Lisa, the intake counselor from an outpatient clinic to arrange speech and physical therapy.

"You really should think about a residential facility," Lisa said after I met her one morning at the rehabilitation ward. "It's not a nursing home, it's a residential treatment center two hours north of Los Angeles that specializes in brain injury. We have attendants around the clock and therapists trained to work with patients who are agitated. There would be someone with Perry 24/7. We just use the nursing home benefits in your insurance to pay for it."

She saw the blank look on my face.

"Look," Lisa said, "this is how insurance works." She sketched a diagram with steps, like a staircase on a yellow legal pad. "You go from hospitalization to acute rehabilitation to a skilled nursing facility, then in-home care. It goes from more intensive medical care to less care. Your insurance covered 30 days of acute rehabilitation here. Your insurance will also cover up to 100 days of a skilled nursing facility, and then in-home services when you get home. If you take Perry home right now, you will lose those 100 days of skilled nursing facility benefits." She crossed off one of the steps with a big X for emphasis. "Your in-home care benefits cover 60 visits only, which you will use up in about four to six weeks. You will lose those 100 days and you won't ever get them back."

Until now, I didn't really understand how health insurance

worked. Neither the social worker or discharge planner at rehabilitation facility had ever explained it to me. If I brought him home now, I would miss out on those 100 days, 100 days that I would not have to be responsible for his care. All this time, I was just thankful that he had survived and woke from his coma. But I knew I was not ready to handle this crazed, agitated person that was emerging. Even though I put on a brave façade to my family and friends, deep down I was terrified. Was I being a coward for looking to place him somewhere for 100 days? And what happened after the 100 days and for the rest of our lives?

"Listen," Lisa said, placing her hand on my arm, "you are in this for the long haul. Brain injury rehab is a long, slow process. You need to figure out how to get the most out of your benefits. Even though Bakersfield is far away, this is what he needs right now. Insurance companies think that the recovery time for brain injury is a year and then they stop coverage."

I stared into her penetrating green eyes that seem to peer inside me and detect the fear lurking there. She exuded calmness and composure in her tailored dark green pantsuit and silk blouse which complemented her olive complexion. I turned around to look at Perry, standing in defiance, surrounded by a nurse and two attendants pleading with him to put his shirt back on. I could see the confusion and panic in his eyes. The prospect of placing him somewhere, anywhere, even if it was far away, didn't seem so daunting now. The truth that I had been avoiding was clear to me in that instant. Everything would not be all right when he got home. Our lives were not going to return to normal. I saw what our lives would be—me, Paul and Zack trying to calm an agitated Perry, coaxing him to put on his clothes, trying to talk rationally to a crazed man— and I didn't want it.

"Okay," I said to Lisa, "what do I need to do to place him there?"

Chapter 9

— ⋙⋘ —

I battled feelings of guilt after making the decision to place Perry in a residential facility. I felt as if I was abandoning Perry by placing him in an institution so far away. What kind of a wife did that make me? His sister cried when I told her about my decision and I was filled with remorse. As the days passed, getting our insurance to pay for the facility proved impossible. I spent days wrangling with intake counselors, doctors and insurance administrators to find out that our insurance would not pay for the facility north of Los Angeles. Our only alternative was to place him at Casa Colina in Pomona, forty-five minutes from our home, which they authorized for 100 days.

I didn't know what to think about placing him there. When it had been mentioned at the rehabilitation hospital, both the discharge planner and the social worker wrinkled their noses and shook their heads. "You don't want to go there."

By their grimaces, I envisioned a scene from *Titicut Follies*, the Frederick Wiseman documentary I saw in college of a naked man in his fifties wailing in a mental institution. But now it was the only alternative available to me and I wondered how bad it would have to be for me to not place him there, in light of his agitation episodes.

Zack, Paul and I went on a hastily arranged tour and were pleasantly surprised by the lobby filled with tall ferns and a stone fireplace, the dining room with pine furniture and blue and white checkered curtains and the physical therapy room with colored mats and levers and pulleys, exercise bikes, parallel bars. A half dozen patients were working with physical therapists, some in wheelchairs, or leg braces. A sense of calm permeated the building. There was no overcrowding, no gray or concrete anywhere, no institutional feel. The patients wore freshly laundered clothing and the therapists were attentive and respectful. Everything looked clean and polished.

I signed the papers for his transfer and on August 15, the date of our 21st wedding anniversary, I had Perry admitted to Casa Colina for 100 days. In previous years, Perry always made a big deal of our anniversary—a special dinner, a surprise gift and always, a dozen long stemmed red roses delivered to me. Even if I was traveling for work or visiting my family, those dozen red roses found me. Last year, on our 20th anniversary, he bought me a three-diamond ring, because when we got married, we had barely scraped up enough money for a thin gold wedding band with tiny diamonds and rubies. "Every time you look at your ring, you will think of me," he said as we admired the way light refracted and sparkled in the center diamond.

This year, I was the only one accompanying him to Casa Colina. Earlier that day, the boys had left for backpacking in the Sierras. They offered to stay with me but I urged them to go. It was their last chance to get to the mountains before Zack left for college and Paul started school again. They needed a break after spending the last two months at the hospital.

As I followed the ambulance on the drive to Casa Colina, my mind was clouded with memories of our wedding day, of our wedding vows, "...for richer, for poorer, in sickness and in health, until death do us part." Had I vowed to take care of him even though his brain was gone? I had read different studies that looked at divorce rates among couples after a spouse suffered a brain injury. The rates ranged from 48% to 78%. I thought about a story I'd read where the wife reported that even though her husband regained most functioning after his brain injury, he was not the man she married. I wondered how different Perry would have to be in order for me to give up my wedding vows. Or would we become one of the divorce statistics?

WHEN WE ARRIVED AT CASA Colina, they unloaded Perry on a gurney. I ran to him as he squinted in the bright sun, disoriented, sweaty and wet from urine.

"Are you okay, Perry?" I asked.

He looked at me and frowned, silent. An attendant greeted us, then ushered me into a conference room.

"I'm going to get him changed and then he will join you," she said. When Perry returned, she sat him at the conference table and said, "It will be just a few minutes and then the speech therapist will come and administer some tests."

Perry was fidgety, he stood and reached for the Post-It notes on the conference table, grabbed pens and tried to scribble on forms. I felt like a mother trying to control a boisterous toddler as I snatched the pens from his hand and coaxed him to sit. I was exhausted and emotionally spent. Where was the help? I wanted to be rid of him, I wanted to escape.

Finally, the speech therapist came and took us to an interview room. After another hour of tests to identify colors on flashcards, then pair alike words and find opposites, they wheeled him to his room. Two attendants were there to help him. *At last*, I thought, *reinforcements to help control him!* I didn't want the responsibility of placating and calming him down. But when they tried to guide him out of the chair to sit on the bed, he looked at them in non-recognition and thrashed his arms. He stood, walked from one bed to the next on unsteady feet, tried to take off his shoes, then his clothes.

I wanted to help him but felt frozen in place, as if I couldn't move. What if they rejected him here, too? Then what would I do?

Margaret, the case manager, walked into the room and saw me watching Perry, tears filling my eyes. She put her arms around me and I began to cry, sobbing into the arms of a total stranger. She patted my back and said, "Let's go back to my office." She guided me out of the room and down the hallway to her office. "This will be a good time to get all the paperwork done." She sat me next to her desk and said, "Your insurance has authorized 100 days and he is going to need all 100 days, I think."

I took a deep breath. One hundred days seemed like a long time. I studied the office while Margaret retrieved forms from her desk drawer. Piles of folders and papers cluttered the surface. To her left, soft-bound books on brain injury and neuropsychology were shoved haphazardly onto the shelves above her computer, their spines and covers bent. On the top shelf of the return sat a skinny, clear vase with six dried up roses, the ribbon tied into a neat bow now a faded dusty red color, the water long evaporated leaving a murky stain. Were they a gift from her husband? What was the occasion for the flowers and why hadn't she thrown them out?

"When he clears from this agitation, we will need to think about options for when he gets home," she said. "You will need to line up 24-hour care."

"But I won't need someone at night, while we are asleep, will we?" I asked. I pictured a nurse wearing a uniform, sitting in the dark, keeping vigil while we slept.

"No, most likely not," she said. "When he goes home, round up all those friends who have offered to help or do something. Ask them to help you watch him one or two hours a week. You are going to need all the help you can get."

I imagined calling his law firm partners in their button-down shirts and gray suits and asking them to watch him for a few hours each day. I wondered what they would do when he became agitated. Would they chat about law while they took him to the bathroom?

"Of course, we need to consider the options if he doesn't clear," she said. "It does happen. I'm not saying he will stay like this forever, but we've had patients that have never cleared from this agitation phase. I just want you to be prepared and to consider all the contingencies."

I could feel sweat in the palms of my hands. I had never considered the possibility that he might not ever emerge from this phase.

"I want you to look into facilities where you could place him, just in case. It's going to be hard to find a place because he's so young. Most places don't take 47 year olds. I know you don't want to hear this right now, but I always feel it's best to be prepared for anything."

I stared at those wilted roses again so that I wouldn't have to meet Margaret's gaze. *If I could just shut my eyes and pretend I was somewhere else, or had some other life than this,* I thought. *I don't want this responsibility. I don't want this life.* I could feel Margaret staring at me, her voice gentle even though she was delivering sobering facts. What was her husband like? It was already 5:00 in the afternoon, the end of the working day. Did he have dinner waiting for her or would she have to cook when she got home? I had no idea what her life was outside of Casa Colina but I envied her life anyway. I desperately wanted some other life. Not this one.

Margaret handed me a thick stack of papers to sign and her cell phone number so that I could call her anytime for updates on Perry's condition.

I WEPT DURING THE FORTY-FIVE minute drive home. Our house was quiet when I stepped through the front door. Only Drake greeted me eagerly with his tail wagging. On the dining room table was the day's mail and a tall vase with a dozen long stemmed red roses. My heart fluttered as I stepped closer. The card read, "With Much Love, Perry" scrawled in Zack's handwriting. I knew the boys meant well in acknowledging our anniversary but after the harrowing day I had, it felt like another stab to my heart. I climbed over the dog gate into the kitchen and curled up on the floor next to Drake, my tears dripping onto his soft fur.

CHAPTER 10

⌇

Two weeks after Perry was transferred to Casa Colina, we left him under the care of his sister Amy so that Paul and I could accompany Zack to drop him off for college. When we arrived in New York, Amy called to say that he had been agitated the night before and it took four attendants to calm him down. I was instantly filled with heartache. Maybe if I had been there, I could have helped him. He always seemed calmer when I was there.

Perry had good days and bad days at Casa Colina. There were times when he was lucid, his eyes came alive with a spark and he would break into a smile at the sight of me. His voice was loud and the words clearly enunciated. He laughed readily at our jokes. I was filled with hope on those days, that enough of him would return and our lives could be somewhat normal. But then there were days when he had the wild-eyed look of non-recognition, of not knowing where he was. He would fidget with his clothes, making motions to pull off his pants. I would have to get the attendants to help him to the bathroom while I fought the urge to escape, to run down the polished linoleum corridors through the lobby to my car and drive away. And now, in New York, I worried about him, yet I felt a sense of relief for not having to witness his agitation and being able to escape into another reality.

But this particular reality, of dropping Zack off at college, was equally distressing. I was releasing Zack into the world, releasing him from my household, from my protective wing. I wouldn't be making him tacos and watching him moan in contentment as he bit into them, or buying him animal crackers with pink and white frosting, or listening for his key to click in the door. I wouldn't find his scribbled lists of tasks he needed to do or his sketchbook with drawings of action figures. I wouldn't know his whereabouts on a daily basis or whether he had eaten or whether he was cold. He had been a rock for me, a voice of reason whenever I doubted myself. How was I going to get through what remained ahead without him?

I sank onto the pillowtop mattress at the W Hotel on Union Square and closed my eyes. I had learned my lesson from our first trip to New York for Zack's orientation and opted for luxury this time. But even in our plush surroundings, I was filled with longing for Perry. Not the agitated Perry who was kicking off his shoes and frowning but the pre-injury Perry with his broad smile and eager embrace. The Perry that would have accompanied me on this trip, that would have laid down beside me and squeezed my hand at this moment and said, "Don't worry, Zack will be fine."

The year before his heart attack, on our 20th wedding anniversary, we had slipped away for the weekend while the boys were at summer camp. It felt glorious to be away, just the two us. We dined in a restaurant overlooking Siletz Bay off the coast of Oregon, our table sprinkled with confetti spelling "Happy Anniversary." Perry smiled at me from across the table.

"These are all distractions, Cyn. Work, raising kids, they are all distractions. When the kids are off to college, when we retire, when it's just you and me again, that's when the fun will begin," he said, raising a glass of champagne in a toast.

I was excited about the prospect of an empty nest, of

spending time alone together again, of reclaiming our private moments before we had children. But now, Perry was in no shape to accompany me anywhere outside of the transitional living center, much less to New York. He wasn't even cognizant enough to know that the day we had planned for all those years ago, of our oldest son leaving for college, was happening right now.

The next morning, after rolling Zack's suitcases four blocks to his dorm room, Paul, Zack and I walked to the Bed Bath & Beyond on Avenue of the Americas. I filled the shopping cart with throw rugs, wash cloths, sheets, comforters, laundry baskets, anything to fill the void of me not being there with Zack. In nine months, when I returned to help him pack to come home for the summer, I would see those throw rugs and wash cloths unused and discarded, but at the time, they filled the emptiness growing inside me.

The moment came at the corner of 3rd Avenue and 14th Street, amid the flashing red numbers on the side of the Virgin Megastore. We couldn't prolong it any longer. We had already bought Zack a printer, scanner, paper and pens, and gone out to dinner. He was anxious to get settled in his dorm. Zack turned to me and I hugged him longer than usual, I didn't want to let go.

I remembered the first three months of his life when I was with him constantly while I stayed home from work, attuned to every rhythm of his body. I loved sitting in the rocking chair with his head perched on my shoulder as I gently rocked, feeling his body go limp with sleep. He had inherited my love of books and art. When he was in elementary school, we anticipated every chapter in the *Indian in the Cupboard* series and wept together at the end of *Sadako and the Thousand Cranes*. As a teenager, we lingered in art museums together, admiring the contrast of light and shadows while Perry and Paul raced through the galleries and waited for us outside. I loved his sense of curiosity and insightful observations. "You smell like graham crackers and sunshine," I would always tell him, as I kissed him good night, inhaling the scent of his hair that reminded me of sheets that had been hung out to dry in the sun.

Eighteen years later on the street in New York, he still smelled like graham crackers and sunshine. My eyes watered and my lips started to quiver.

"Goodbye, Zack," I managed to choke out.

"You take care of yourself, Mom," he whispered into my ear. "Don't worry about me. I'll be fine and you're going to be okay, too."

As he said his goodbye to Paul, I wanted to wail at the top of my lungs. I stood still, watching Zack's long black hair until he disappeared into the crowd, his figure bobbing with the fast New York stride he had already acquired. I wanted to get swallowed into the streets of New York too, away from what awaited me in Los Angeles. But then I felt a hand on my elbow, a squeeze on my shoulder as tears streamed down my cheeks.

"Come on, Mom, let's go see a movie," said Paul.

I let myself be guided down Third Avenue into a Cineplex, wiping tears from my eyes. As I sat in the dark, my tears flowed. I let myself be lost in the *Pirates of the Caribbean* while swords clashed and waves heaved. I let myself forget, for the moment, about brain injury and first-born sons going off to college.

CHAPTER 11

꧁

During Perry's stay at Casa Colina there was no pattern to his behavior. There was no way of predicting what his state of mind would be when we visited. In his lucid moments, I saw glimpses of the former Perry, his sparkling eyes full of love, his Cheshire Cat smile with a sign of mischief, the arching of his brows and his deep, nasally voice. Whenever one of the attendants pointed to me and asked him, "Who's she?" he would always break into a smile and say the same thing: "My beautiful wife, Cynthia." But in his agitated moments, I didn't know who he was. There was a hardness in his eyes, a disconnection that made him appear as a stranger to me. He was lost in silence and unresponsive, frowning.

I hated the unpredictability of his behavior. I hated the uncertainty of our future. I hated the long drive to Pomona. It often took more than an hour, sometimes up to ninety minutes. It was my only moment of solitude and during those moments, away from Paul's watchful eye and the facade of strength I kept in front of my coworkers, I cried for my old life. I longed to have my genial companion back who was conversant, considerate, and made me laugh. I didn't care about the lawyering and the cocktail parties and the chatter about European vacations and private schools. I wanted to be able to travel with him again, to hike in the wilderness, to see a movie, have my secret smiles and hand squeezes. I longed for Perry's laughter and gentleness with every nerve in my body.

I cried as I replayed the scene at the Benson Hotel over and over in my mind. Why did I go blank, why didn't I remember the lesson from twelve years earlier when Perry and I attended a CPR class at the kids' elementary school? The dummy's lips were worn and the rubber body sticky from wear, but we learned how to do chest compressions, count, press again. We giggled through the class, what did we know back then about emergencies and heart attacks? We were in our mid-30s Perry had just made partner at his law firm and I was a stay-at-home mom. Our boys were enrolled in private school, we had bought our first home. The future was bright and promising. Why didn't we take that course more seriously?

I cried when I remembered the words of the cardiologist in Portland, "...because no resuscitation was initiated, and I'm not blaming you for not performing CPR, your husband had no oxygen flowing to his brain and may have suffered brain damage." But didn't he really mean that it was my fault? Why didn't I start CPR? Couldn't I have just done a few chest compressions to get blood to his brain?

I cried when I thought of our future, for the vacations still to be planned, for our dreams to grow old and retire together. I cried for the loss of my companion, my sounding board, my source of security and comfort. I cried because I didn't feel whole without Perry, he was like my right arm, an appendage attached to me, the opinion I always valued and trusted. I cried because I didn't have anyone to tell me I was smart when I was filled with doubt.

I cried when I thought about the broken sprinkler on the front lawn and when the kitchen lights flickered for no reason and we lost power. I cried when I thought of our dog Drake, waiting patiently for someone to walk him, hoping that Perry would appear.

I cried when he didn't recognize his favorite Shimano fly fishing reel and gold colored spinning reel. Perry had loved his fishing equipment. Before he went out on his boat, he would spend hours in the garage fussing with his lines, rods and reels. He used to call me from work, excited about the latest purchase.

"Cyn, I just ordered this really nice Shimano fly fishing reel. It's a big one and I can use it for saltwater fly fishing. What do you think?"

"Sounds good to me," I said, not knowing the difference between a fly fishing reel for saltwater or freshwater, or why this one was so special.

But when I brought him that reel at Casa Colina, he didn't recognize the purple felt bag. He took out the reel and held it in his palm, his face puzzled. He ran his stubby fingers over the cut-out holes in the reel, then turned it over. He stared at it, silent.

"It's your special Shimano reel," I said. "Do you remember when you bought it and how excited you were?"

"No," he said, slowly turning it in his hands. With the weight he lost during his coma, the tops of his hands seemed more wrinkled and freckled. He put the Shimano reel on the desk.

"What about this one?" I asked, handing him the other reel. He pulled the spool into place, then cranked it one turn.

"It's a spinning reel," he whispered, "for fishing with a lure or bait." He set it down on the desk, disinterested then turned away. In that moment, it seemed that all hope was lost.

"Oh, Perry," I pleaded in the darkness, peering out the windshield through my tears. "Come back to me. I need you, I can't handle this on my own."

I felt like a widow, but Perry wasn't dead. I was mourning the loss of someone who was still alive, albeit in a different form. This was an entirely different type of grief. And during those times, I longed for the comfort of religion. I thought of the healing prayer that Perry's cousins had sang in Hebrew while he was in intensive care. I had squirmed when I heard the unfamiliar Hebrew words and didn't know if I should bow my head or look up. Neither Perry nor I was deeply religious. But the Hebrew phrases became comforting to me.

"Retaeinu Adonay V'Nerafeh, Hosheeinu v'nerasheinu kee Tehilateinu Atah."

Heal us, oh God, and we shall be healed.

I would sing to myself when I left the hospital in the evenings. Something about the cadence and melody resonated with me. I felt a sense of spirituality, a connection with an ancient tradition. And now, mourning for the old Perry and our old life, I longed for a formal ritual, a way to say goodbye to his former self. I wanted to sing a liturgy at a Catholic funeral mass, recite Kaddish in Hebrew, receive visitors while sitting Shiva or light incense and pray in his memory in a Buddhist temple.

I WONDERED IF I COULD adapt to the new Perry and love him in the same way. I thought about what there was that still remained to love and how bad would it have to get for me to stop loving him. What remained of a marriage if shared memories were lost? I had read that in most brain injury cases, short-term memory was the first to go, whereas long term memory generally stayed intact. Memories that occurred right before the event were usually lost. I quizzed him on what he could remember.

"Do you remember our trip to Prague and Vienna?" I asked. We had gone there for spring break, three months before his heart attack.

"Not really," he said.

"How about your fishing trip to La Paz?" He had taken that trip a month before his heart attack, with Paul and our neighbor Manny.

"Not really."

"What about Zack's graduation?" The high school graduation occurred the week before his heart attack.

He looked at me without a hint of recognition.

"What do you remember?" I asked.

"I remember going to law school and working really hard. I remember taking the bar exam and passing. I remember my law firm," he said, his voice fading to a whisper. "I remember how much I love you."

CHAPTER 12

―◆―

As summer gave way to fall and the stifling heat cooled to crisp, clear days, my responses to Perry's condition flattened; I didn't jump for joy during his alert and lucid moments. I knew that every upward moment would be accompanied by an equally low moment, when I would feel despair again. Grief invaded my body like a virus, attacking every muscle that ached with longing for our former lives.

There were days when everything in my life seemed broken and I wanted to give up and walk away. The oven would not warm up or the circuit breakers would not reset or the runners on Paul's dresser broke, so we couldn't close the drawers. One morning, I stepped into the backyard to take out the garbage and noticed that the dog waste had not been picked up. It was Paul's main job: walk the dog and pick up his waste before the gardener came on Thursdays. Angry, I went into the house and got a plastic bag to pick it up. *How many days had he let this go?* I thought, as the bag began to fill. I put down the shovel to tie up the bag but the bottom broke, littering my black work shoes with dog turds. I went back in the house for another plastic bag, cleaned up again then stormed back into the kitchen.

"God damn it, Paul! Why didn't you clean up in the backyard?" I yelled. "How hard could it be?"

Paul came out of his room, apologetic.

"Sorry, Mom, I was too tired yesterday," he said.

We were running late, there was no time for breakfast. I grabbed my purse and coffee and went out to the car, fighting back tears. *I can't do this. I hate my life.*

Paul joined me in the car, silent. Tears slid down my checks as we headed toward his school. I didn't want this life anymore, but what alternatives did I have? Divorce Perry and leave him in an assisted living facility? Run away from Zack and Paul and let them fend for themselves? All I could do was endure this living hell.

"I'm sorry Mom, I know you're under a lot of stress," Paul said.

"I just don't understand why you can't pick up the dog poo. How hard is that? Just once a week, how hard can it be? The only thing I ask of you is to walk the dog and pick up after him," I yelled, through clenched teeth.

"I know, I know! I said I was sorry!" He let out a sob as his face dissolved into tears. "I'm hurting too, you know. I hate my life! I'm not a carefree kid anymore! I have a brain damaged father!"

I knew he was hurting as much as I was. I saw the sadness in his face, his quietness at home when we had dinner together. When he was with me at Casa Colina, I could see the impatience in his eyes as they darted around the room. I knew he wanted to be somewhere else, anywhere but Casa Colina. That fall, a group of mothers from his school delivered meals to him on the nights that I was in Pomona. I knew how awkward it was for him to have to interact with other mothers that he didn't know and accept food from them as if he was a charity case. Everything in his life had changed, too.

As we approached his school, I didn't make the left hand turn toward the drop-off spot. I continued on for a few blocks and pulled into the parking lot of a restaurant where we both cried, reaching for the box of Kleenex in the back.

"My life is miserable, too," I said through my tears. I thought of all the times I tried not to cry in front of Paul, how I felt I needed to stay strong for him. I reached for his arm in an attempt to comfort him. His eyes were closed as he tilted his head back, his mouth in a grimace. "We need to find ways to help each other," I said. "Let's make sure we take time out for ourselves." But even as I said those words, it sounded hollow. There was nothing I could do to ease Paul's pain and sorrow. Everything in our lives was broken and there wasn't a way to fix it.

I wished we could just get on the freeway and drive east to join Zack in New York where he was having a blast, or north to the comfort of my family—away from Los Angeles, away from Pomona, away from brain injury. Instead, I started the car again, dropped Paul off at school and headed toward downtown on the freeway.

Most days, I was able to keep a calm front as I faced a constant stream of well-wishers who wanted to know about Perry's progress and how I was doing. One work acquaintance would corner me in the most public of places, in a crowded elevator or in a line for a shuttle bus and ask in his booming voice, "How is Perry doing?"

I would explain in low tones, "He's fine, he's walking, he's talking, he's working with therapists." What else can be said in a crowded elevator where the norm is to stare at your feet or the ceiling, silent? How could I say, *"He's fucked up! He needs help bathing, going to the bathroom, dressing!"*

Another acquaintance once pressed her hand on my arm and said, "God doesn't give you more than you can handle," trying to reassure me. I wanted to slap her hand away and say, *"That's the stupidest thing I ever heard. What kind of God unleashes this kind of hell on someone?"*

And then there was Perry's eighty-year-old Uncle Ralph who called every few weeks demanding a progress report.

He never asked how I was coping or how the boys were. "Call me back and let me know the latest developments in Perry's case," he would order, in his bellowing tone, on our answering machine. When I did reach him by phone, he always said, "He was such a successful attorney and now this ... Is he going to be able to return to work? How are you going to pay for college?" I dreaded his calls. When I reported that Perry had improved, he asked, "Do you mean he will be able to work again?" and then moan in disappointment when I said it wasn't likely.

But there were also acts of kindness, such as the wife of my former boss, who looked at me with concern and then wrung her hands when we met at a reception. "I am so sorry. It's so tragic and I feel for you. I don't know what the right thing is to say but I just want you to know that I think about you and Perry all the time."

I was comforted; it was just the right thing to say.

There were days when I moved in robotic motions of sorrow, a walking collection of nerves and pain. My eyes seem to rest in a constant well of tears ready to spill at any moment. Those were the days I wanted to hide in my cubicle, work on numbers and not talk to anyone. But on one of those days, I had to drive to the San Fernando Valley and make a presentation for new principals on using our data systems. As I drove toward the freeway on-ramp downtown, I glimpsed the Gas Company Tower where Perry's law firm was housed. I pictured Perry in his gray suit, walking across Figueroa to meet me for lunch, the bounce in his step as he crossed the street, the ever-ready smile when he got within sight of me. I felt a lurch in my stomach, a tightening of muscles as a surge of longing washed over me.

In the meeting room in the valley, Cindy, my colleague had already set up the projector and passed out the materials. As the room began to fill, I felt myself weaken. *I can't do this. I'm not up for this.* I wanted to be at home, in bed, curled in a fetal position.

"I'll do the first part," said Cindy. Maybe she sensed the sadness in me, maybe she could see misery oozing from my pores.

I nodded and walked into the empty room next door, then stared out the window. Perhaps I needed to take an extended leave from work. But what would my life be filled with instead? I tried to picture myself at Casa Colina all day, following Perry from one therapy appointment to the next, being his constant cheerleader, urging him to remember, to focus, to walk. What kind of life would that be?

But how could I continue to function in this manner, handling work, visiting him at Casa Colina, taking care of Paul and all other household chores? Why didn't I just have someone else take over this training? The principals in the Valley were always tough and they always asked hard questions, challenged the presenter. *How can I do this?* I thought about my mother and stiffened. *No, I don't want to be like my mother. I can do this.* I remembered what Perry used to tell me whenever I got stressed, "The only way to get rid of stress is to tackle it head on. Just chip away at all the things that are nagging at you and get them done, one by one." I could hear him telling me, "You can do it, Cyn, you are smart and capable." I took a deep breath. I needed to focus on the things I could control and just get through them, one by one. The first was getting through this presentation.

In the other room, I heard applause. Cindy was done and it was time for my part. I straightened my blouse and jacket, then walked into the room and faced the audience. They looked at me, expectant. I forced a smile on my face and heard my voice shake and quiver as I introduced myself. But when I got to the part about how to examine data and the data inquiry cycle, I could feel my face and body relaxing. *I know this stuff. I can do this.* Heads nodded in agreement, the audience was engaged as I moved around the room, gesticulating, in my element now, my shoulders loose and free of tension. I had the participants count off to split into smaller groups for discussion, then I moved around the room, listening, answering questions. The image of Perry in his gray suit faded, my pain and sorrow faded. I had control of the room and I was comfortable. *I can get through this.*

CHAPTER 13

—\l/—

In October, it was Parent Day at Paul's school, the first time I had ever attended one without Perry. All morning, I had listened to other parents chatter about AP Exams and driving permits but my mind was on Perry. We had started his transition to home with day visits. I had gone through a mixture of relief and panic at the thought of bringing him home. Relief because I would no longer have to drive to Pomona but panic over what his state of mind would be at the time of discharge. I had taken him on short drives around Pomona, getting used to being in a car with him again. On his first visit home, he recognized the house and had looked so peaceful, so relaxed, without a hint of brain injury or agitation when he napped on our bed. I could picture a semblance of normal family life once again.

But being at Parent Day without Perry reminded me that we didn't have a normal family life and that our lives were now totally different. I leaned against a wall near the refreshment table and hoped that no one would approach me or ask me questions. Then I spotted Adrianna. She saw me at the same time and we began moving towards each other, dodging through the throngs of parents. Trim in her denim jacket and oversized beige scarf, her straight brown hair was pulled into a tight ponytail. I could see the lines of concern on her face as she reached out her arms to give me a bear hug.

"Are you okay?" she said, squeezing me tight. I hugged her back. Over the years, our sons had spent lots of time together and I had always wanted to get to know her better but we didn't move in the same social circles.

"So, what happened?" she asked.

I stepped back to face her. "We were in Portland for a bar mitzvah, just for the night," I said. "Perry had a heart attack and his heart stopped. He didn't get enough oxygen to his brain and now he has brain damage."

"But why? Why did he lose oxygen to his brain?" She shook her head in disbelief. "Where were you? Weren't you right there?"

I paused. Was she blaming me?

"They couldn't resuscitate him," I said. "I was right there."

But she was already looking away, having spotted another mother to connect with. It was time for the next class and I moved away, not knowing what to say. *I was right there*, I wanted to tell her, *but it happened so fast. I was paralyzed. I was helpless.*

Adrianna's comment pierced me with guilt again and haunted me for weeks and months to come. I couldn't even concentrate on the rest of the classes I attended. My mind kept playing the questions over and over: *Was it my fault? Why didn't I start CPR right away?*

When I got home, I immediately went to Paul's bedroom where he was sitting on his bed, listening to music.

"Was it my fault that I didn't do CPR? Could I have done something?"

"You can't keep thinking about the past, Mom," said Paul, removing the headphones from his ears. "We just have to move forward. What happened, happened. You can't change it."

Later that weekend, I called Zack in New York. "I feel terrible. She asked me why your dad didn't get enough oxygen to his brain, as if she was accusing me of not doing something. Was she right? Was it my fault?"

I heard him take a deep breath. "Don't even go there," said Zack. "Don't get upset by Adrianna. She wasn't there and she doesn't know. Don't play the 'what if' game. It won't get you anywhere and it will only make you feel worse."

But I couldn't block out the remorse. Why didn't I insist we drive to the hospital when he first complained of pain? I made him walk with me to Powell's bookstore even though he had to stop to buy Rolaids. In the emergency room in Oregon, the cardiologist said it was most likely the clogging of his artery that was giving him pain, not heartburn.

Where could I direct my sense of guilt? I longed for absolution, to lock myself into a confessional box and unleash my sins, ask for forgiveness, express my sorrow. I wanted to receive my penance, to say I was sorry for what I had not done and make amends. I wanted a priest to absolve me and tell me to go in peace. I wanted the comfort of a higher power even though I was still conflicted about whether I truly believed in God.

ONE EVENING, AFTER ATTENDING A class on wilderness medicine, Paul burst through the door. "You know Mom, there was nothing you could have done. CPR does not revive someone with ventricular fibrillation."

I put down the book I was reading and looked at him.

"What?" I asked. "What is ventricular fibrillation? I thought he had a heart attack."

"He did and it sent his heart into some kind of arrhythmia, then he went into ventricular fibrillation," he said. "Don't you remember the cardiologist telling us that after he put in the stent?"

I had dim memories of what was said that night in Portland. I remembered the cardiologist showing us a scan of Perry's heart with squiggly lines. But Paul heard and remembered everything, just like he did when he was eight and we bought our minivan. He had paid close attention when the salesman went through all the features while the rest of us were distracted. He was the one who knew where the spare tire was stored and how to fold back the rear seat.

I sent for Perry's medical records from Portland and scanned through pages of case notes, printouts of his heart rhythms and lab tests. On the intake form, "myocardial infarction and subsequent ventricular fibrillation" were listed under principal diagnosis. I researched "ventricular fibrillation," a condition in which the heart's electrical activity becomes disordered, where blood is not removed from the heart. Ventricular fibrillation caused unconsciousness in seconds and sudden cardiac death follows in minutes unless medical help is provided immediately.

My heart rate quickened. Maybe my presence in the room that night in Portland hadn't hurt Perry; maybe it had actually helped him. What if we hadn't been together in a hotel room at 11:00 that night in Portland? If we'd been at home, what were the odds we would have been in the same room? Perry was an early bird, often asleep in bed by 11:00 while I tended to stay up late reading or watching TV in the living room. I would not have been there to hear his gasp and reach for the phone. If I hadn't been right next to him, he could have easily died that night. Help would have come too late.

In all of the articles I read about ventricular fibrillation, CPR was recommended as immediate treatment but electric shock from a defibrillator was the only treatment that would restore a normal heartbeat. Survival rates for ventricular fibrillation were rare outside of hospitals and ranged from two percent to twenty-five percent. The doctors in Portland had given him a fifteen percent chance for survival. He could have easily slipped away that night in Portland.

I imagined my life without him, a future filled with longing, like the longing I had for my father when he died. The memory of my father's hugs, when he gathered me in his arms and I felt the cold night air on his tweed jacket when he walked into the house from the garage stayed with me for years. The longing never stopped.

I began reading the obituary page of the newspaper every day, carefully combing through each of the squares in tiny font detailing who had passed, noting when they were born, how old they were at death. I studied the ones that died young, in their 40s or 50s and lingered over the ones that listed "heart attack" as the cause of death. I wondered about their survivors. Did they blame the doctors, did they administer CPR? I pictured their lives, bereft, empty without their husband, or wife or mother or father, filled with an entirely different type of pain than mine. I was grateful to still have Perry with me, I could hold him, touch him, kiss him. A life without him would be much worse.

Was there something we could have done to detect this earlier? If only I had made him go back to the doctor. Three months before his heart attack, he complained of heartburn and saw his primary care doctor. She didn't do an EKG, or order a stress test that could have possibly revealed the blockage in his artery. Instead, she sent him home with a prescription for acid reflux, with instructions to stay away from tomatoes, onions, peppers and chocolate to avoid heartburn.

One article pointed out the difficulty in knowing when a person would be prone to ventricular fibrillation and how to assess the risks because the symptoms were often confused with indigestion and heartburn. Even people with no previous risk factors were felled by sudden cardiac arrest. I felt some sense of relief after reading these articles but still, Adrianna's comment haunted me, the guilt lingered. It would never entirely go away.

LATER THAT MONTH, WE BEGAN the first of several overnight visits to ease us into Perry's eventual discharge home. On his first overnight visit, his sister was visiting and Perry joined in the laughter around the dinner table. We watched a movie in the living room and he was alert and attentive. But when we went to bed that night, he laid in bed stiff and tense. Then he began moving restlessly, kicking off the blankets, sometimes sitting up or trying to stand.

"What's the matter, Perry?" I asked. "Do you need something?"

He didn't respond to my questions but kept up his restless movements. At three in morning, I took him to the bathroom and he relieved himself. Back in bed, he finally fell asleep but I was still awake, listening to his soft snoring and on edge, attuned to his every move, every twitch.

The next morning, he was hard to rouse and didn't want to get up. I let him sleep until 9:00, then 9:30. He was dazed and unresponsive when I woke him and tried to get him in a sitting position. In the shower, I poured shampoo into the palm of his hand, but instead of spreading it on his head as I cued him, he rubbed it between his fingers until it was gone. I handed him the soap and he held it in his hand, unmoving. After I soaped and rinsed him off, he stood still, inert and in a daze, not making any effort to follow my cues. When I tried to get his sweatpants on him, he wouldn't lift his leg so I could slip them over his feet.

"Move your foot, Perry," I said.

He stood still as a statue, feet firmly planted. I lifted his left foot, then his right and realized how hard it was to get him dressed when he didn't cooperate. He stared at his reflection in the mirror when I spread shaving cream on his face and wouldn't hold the razor in his hand. After I got him dressed, he walked back to the bedroom, climbed into bed and closed his eyes. It took me and Paul to pull him into a sitting position, then onto his feet to walk to the dining table for breakfast. He ate if we fed him but otherwise made no effort to lift his spoon with cereal.

I got up from the table, went into the bathroom, closed the door then held my head in my hands and cried.

My God, what has he turned into? I thought. *What am I going to do when he gets home? Do I have the strength and patience to do this?*

I thought about Margaret's insistence that I have a back-up plan, an assisted living facility in case this didn't work out. Maybe she was right. When it was time to take Perry back to Casa Colina the next day, I was relieved.

A FEW WEEKS LATER, WE brought him home for a second overnight visit. This time, he was alert and responsive. We had dinner across the street with our neighbors. Although he didn't initiate speech, he followed along with the conversation, his eyes aware and curious, laughing at the appropriate parts. At home before bed, his eyes were clear, his expression serious.

"I don't know where I belong," he said. "It feels strange."

"What feels strange?" I asked.

"Me," he said. "I have trouble with spatial relationships."

Before I could probe further, he closed his eyes and sank into a deep sleep. He slept soundly through the night, without twitching or waking.

The next morning, I woke feeling rested from my uninterrupted sleep. I got up before he woke and showered and dressed, ready to face the challenge of his morning routine. I went into the bedroom and pulled up the shades to let in the morning light.

"Time to get up, Perry, good morning!" I said, turning to face him.

He opened his eyes and a smile lit his face at the sight of me, his brown eyes lively and full of love. I pulled the comforter back, then the sheets. I guided his legs to the edge of the bed, directed his feet to the floor, then pulled him up to a sitting position to make it easier for him to stand. I waited until he gained his balance, then held his hand as we walked slowly through the hallway to the long, narrow bathroom. He lathered his own hair with shampoo after I poured it into his hand. After his shower, I toweled him off and positioned him in front of the sink. I squeezed toothpaste on his toothbrush and guided his hand to his mouth. He brushed lightly, then set the toothbrush on the counter. I followed up with more rigorous brushing and filled his cup with water. He took a big sip, swished and spit out. I smeared shaving cream on my fingers, spread it on his cheeks. I placed the razor in his hand and he took a few feeble strokes on one side of his face, then the other, then his chin. He handed me the razor and I shaved the spots he missed. I pulled his polo shirt over his head and he reached his arms through the sleeves. He lifted his leg, first the right, then the left as I guided them into his sweatpants. I placed the hairbrush in his hand and he combed the wispy tuft of brown hair on the top of his head, then the sides over his ears. He studied his reflection in the mirror with raised eyebrows and smiled, then turned to look at me.

"You look so handsome!" I told him and he laughed, pursed his lips for a kiss. I reached to hug him and inhaled his scent, a mixture of Tide detergent, Caress soap, shaving cream and musky sweat, as I pressed my face onto his shoulder. His arms folded me into a familiar embrace. He smelled the same and I was grateful that he was still here. This was my absolution.

CHAPTER 14

⁓⁓⁓

On the Friday before Thanksgiving, Perry was discharged home. I felt a sense of relief as I drove away from Casa Colina, the car loaded with his clothes, posters, pictures, boom box and TV. I could sleep in on weekends. I could cook again. For the past 100 days, my life had been divided between the hospital and home. I never felt as if I was fully present at either place. When I was at Casa Colina, I worried about Paul and Zack in college. When I was at home, my thoughts were consumed by Perry.

The very next morning, on a Saturday, Ginger, an occupational therapist from our in-home and community care agency, arrived to orient us to Perry's new routine. She began by describing what I needed to do. "Make sure that there is structure to his days," she said. "You will need a daily journal to write down his activities and schedule each day. Whoever is with him, don't let him sit around the house and watch TV all day. He needs activities, he needs stimulation."

I felt a knot forming in my stomach. All this time I had been so focused on the fact that he was alive that I didn't grasp the full impact of my situation. His being home meant that I was responsible for keeping him engaged and active every minute of the day. Perry could not be left alone. In that moment, I understood what 24-hour care meant. I could not leave the house to take Paul to school or make a quick trip to the grocery store or browse in a bookstore without finding someone to stay with him. I had lost all of my personal freedom.

How lightly I had treated those days when Perry was at Casa Colina. Paul and I had developed a new routine. Whenever I felt overwhelmed, he would suggest that we go out to eat or to a movie. Out went our old rules about prescribed bed times on school nights as we stayed up late watching TV. Now, everything would have to change with Perry home.

"You will need to transfer all his medications to your local pharmacy, then you want to get a pill organizer to help you keep track of which ones he takes in the morning and which ones in the evening," Ginger continued.

I gulped. This was going to be my responsibility, too. I had no medical training and wasn't sure what I should be watchful of in terms of his medical condition. There wasn't going to be an army of resident technicians to help me, there would be no medical staff to ask questions to whenever I felt unsure of his care. It was all up to me.

"What did he like to do on weekends?" asked Ginger. "What kinds of things could we work on? Cooking? Gardening?"

I paused. Before his brain injury, we were always together, running errands, chauffeuring the boys to their various sports or school events. Our lives had seemed so hectic and crowded with obligations. What did he do that was his only and didn't involve me? He liked to cook elaborate dinners when we entertained but wasn't much of a daily cook. He had no interest in gardening except when I needed his muscle power to pull out a stubborn root.

"He loves to fish and has a boat in the marina. He liked to ride his bike to the beach. He liked to tinker around the house and repair things," I said before realizing that these things were probably lost to him now. I needed to think of what he could do now, in his current state. "He walked the dog."

Ginger nodded. "We can go for walks in the neighborhood. One last thing—get him used to being out in public but be careful that he doesn't get overstimulated. A lot of brain injury patients get overwhelmed in large crowds and it may lead to agitation. There's just too much information to take in at one time."

The knot in my stomach grew. How big was a large crowd? What will happen at Christmas when my family clan of thirty gathered? Did that mean that we could no longer go to parties? What about flying in airplanes or our season tickets for the Dodgers and the Hollywood Bowl?

THE FOLLOWING WEEK I STAYED home from work to orientate the caregiver and Perry. Weeks earlier, Paul and I had interviewed caregivers from an agency, one Filipino man after the other. I wasn't even sure what we should be asking in those interviews, other than what their experience was with brain injury and how they handled agitation. As we met each prospective caregiver, I tried to imagine him in our home, a part of our daily life and a constant presence at the dining table. We settled on Rafael, a mild-mannered, fit man in his twenties who seemed self-assured. He had even spent time with Perry at Casa Colina before his discharge so he could get used to his caregiving routine.

On Monday morning at 7:00 a.m., I waited for the Rafael to arrive. The minutes passed, 7:15, then 7:30. I searched through my piles of paper to find his cell phone number and called. He answered after four rings.

"Oh, I didn't know I was supposed to come today," he said. "I'll leave right now but I won't get there until 8:30. I live in Glendale."

I looked at my watch. I needed to leave at 7:45 to get Paul to school by 8:00. There was no way he could be here on time. I needed to get Paul to school in the next fifteen minutes. I called Nancy across the street to stay with Perry while I raced to get Paul to school.

By the time Rafael arrived, I had already showered and dressed Perry and was feeding him breakfast. There were no therapists scheduled that day. I sat at the dining room table watching Perry spoon cereal to his mouth and wondered how I was going to fill the day. I couldn't just let him sit on the couch all day with the caregiver sitting next to him. I didn't feel comfortable leaving them at the dining table while I read a book on the living room couch or went into the den to surf the Internet. I couldn't help feeling like a hostess, asking Rafael if he wanted water or a snack. I needed to direct his activities and keep both Rafael and Perry in motion, but how?

We finally went for a walk in the neighborhood, the three of us crowded on the sidewalk, flanking Perry while he moved slowly with his stutter step. When we got home, only one hour had elapsed. I tried to think of other tasks to fill up the time. We went to the drugstore to buy pill organizers, then the office supply store for binders and dividers, then had lunch out. When we got home it was only mid-afternoon. How could time move so slowly? Before his heart attack, there never seemed to be enough hours to run our errands, pick up children and then cook dinner. Now the hours yawned open in front of us and I didn't know how to fill them. I was relieved when it was 3:00 and we could all go out again to pick up Paul from school.

The next morning, the phone rang at 7:15. It was Rafael.

"My car won't start. I'm waiting for someone to come to see what's wrong. I won't be able to make it at 8:00. I'm very sorry."

I hung up the phone and panicked. It was just like when the boys were toddlers and I was still working. The sitter always had car trouble and Perry and I would try to rearrange our schedules so that we could take turns staying with the boys. Now I didn't have anyone to juggle schedules with. What would happen next week when I had to get to work? I thought about all the future days when I would have early morning meetings or appointments. For the first time, the thought entered my mind that maybe I would not be able to carry on my career.

I wondered how I was going to get Paul to school. I couldn't impose on Nancy again and ask her to stay. I hustled Perry out of bed, changed him into a pair of sweatpants and a tee shirt, not bothering to brush his teeth or shower him. We helped him into the van and drove Paul to school.

When I got home, I called the agency.

"Where is our caregiver?" I yelled. "For two days in a row, I have not had anyone here at 8:00. This is not working out!"

They apologized profusely and promised to send a replacement caregiver. I hung up the phone and cried. *I can't do this.* The responsibility of caring for Perry was too much. *I can't do this on my own.*

A few hours later, Leonard, the replacement caregiver arrived. Short and wiry, he had an easy smile and a relaxed air of assurance. He looked straight at Perry and spoke to him in a normal voice, not in an exaggerated tone reserved for children like some caregivers did or in a hesitant manner. By the end of the week, we decided to keep Leonard moving forward.

The in-home care agency also sent Cat, the physical therapist, who demonstrated strategies for us to use to improve Perry's walking and balance. "Practice these every day," she said as she taught us how to make Perry shout our names, then toss us a beach ball to increase his verbal skills. She showed us how to point out landmarks on our walks in the neighborhood as she kept up her steady chatter.

There was Mike, the speech therapist, who showed us warm up exercises where Perry said "AHHHH" and held it for 15 to 20 seconds. "It helps loosen the vocal cords," he said. "You should do this with him daily." Then he placed Perry in front of the computer to work on a concentration game using software for brain injured patients. "I'm going to leave you these disks," he said. "You can have him practice this daily, too."

By the end of that first week, I was exhausted by the sheer number of activities and strategies that we were supposed to be doing with Perry. Each event had to be logged and tracked in his memory journal. Overwhelmed, I just wanted to sit on the couch and read a magazine. But as I walked through the house, Paul was watching TV in the living room. In the kitchen, Virginia, our housekeeper who picked up Paul afterschool and helped with household chores, was emptying the dishwasher. I walked into the den but Leonard and Perry were doing their voice exercises on the back porch. I listened to them saying "AHHHH," and felt tense and unsettled. I had always felt that my home was the one place I could retreat from the world and unwind. But now our house felt invaded by all the helpers and therapists. I had no sanctuary, no place of refuge. All those months at the hospital, rehabilitation center and residential facility were just a prelude to this—adapting my life to 24-hour care. My life was no longer my own.

CHAPTER 15

–⁣\⁣⁄⁣–

Months before his discharge from Casa Colina, the case manager had suggested that I file for conservatorship.

"It's relatively easy," she said. "I have clients that have done it on a temporary basis. You just need to consult an attorney."

But I resisted. I wasn't ready to face the reality of disability and conservatorship yet. Something deep inside me resisted the entire notion. My images of people needing conservatorship were elderly or infirm clients with no family, not someone like Perry. Was it really necessary?

I turned to Perry's law firm for advice. They would know what to do and what the best path forward was. But they didn't handle conservatorship issues and had no advice to offer. They did assign me a young, bubbly associate to help me find a suitable firm. When I met with her in a conference room on the 40th floor of their downtown office, I was overcome by wistfulness. I looked out the window to suburbs draped in brown smog east of downtown. It was the same view Perry used to have from his office window. I studied the polished wood table, the chairs with chrome accents, and the real artwork on the walls. All of this was now lost to us—the status account for half of all your income and assets. It doesn't make sense unless you are involved in real estate transactions. I recommend that you wait and see what happens in the recovery process."

I left Marc's office feeling relieved. He was on my side, he was my ally. He didn't think it was necessary. Conservatorship seemed so extreme, to have him declared legally incompetent would mean that I was giving up any hope of recovery, of improvement, that he was truly damaged beyond repair. I wasn't ready to accept that.

A MONTH LATER, I WAS still waiting for Perry's disability insurance claim to be approved. Payments were scheduled to begin in January. I had read through his policy and calculated the amount. It was less than his income as a working partner but was enough to support our lifestyle, even with the amount that we paid for caregiving. However, it was already December and we had not heard from the insurance company. We had money in savings, but needed the disability payments for our monthly expenses. When I called they told me they were waiting for his medical report. When I pressed for details, they said they weren't authorized to give me any more information since I was not the claimant. I was getting nervous. I called the benefits administrator for the firm.

"Can you help me out?" I asked. "What can I do to get payments started?"

Two days later she called back. "I'm sorry, the insurance company says they need a conservator for Perry before they make payments. There's nothing we can do until you file for conservatorship."

I didn't remember reading anything about a conservatorship requirement in the insurance policy. I immediately called Marc and told him we needed to reopen the case.

"Wow, this is going to take some time. They are waiting for this to occur before they issue payments to you?" he asked. "It may be a few weeks before we can even schedule a court hearing. Do you have enough money to tide you over if it takes a couple of months?"

"Yes," I said, but I started to worry. What if took longer than a couple of months or if they denied benefits? Then what would we do?

The next day, Marc's paralegal called with a list of questions: the value of Perry's estate, the names and addresses of Perry's siblings, parents and children, current assets and bank accounts. "I'm also going to secure a bond and I'll try to get the minimum of $6,000. Keep all your receipts. You will need to open a special account just for the disability payments for better accounting." My head was swimming from all the details.

"I still think this is highly unusual. I've never had a case where a disability insurance company has insisted on conservatorship in a case like this. Besides, most of the cases I handle, the clients are deteriorating, rather than slowly getting better, like your husband," Marc said to me over the phone later in the day. "Do you have an advocate at the firm that I can talk to?"

I connected Marc with Rich at the law firm. Together, they questioned the authority of the disability insurance company to demand conservatorship. Their query was escalated to the director of benefits administration at the law firm headquarters in Chicago. The law firm directed their demand straight to the General Counsel for the disability insurance company. The demands from so many attorneys must have gotten someone at the insurance company nervous. Within days, we were notified that payments would begin immediately and were not conditional upon conservatorship.

I felt like breaking out into a victory dance. At least there was one piece of my life I was able to preserve for now.

CHAPTER 16

_ \/ _

As Christmas approached, I wondered if Perry would be able to handle my family's annual get together. For the past five years, my family had gathered at Seascape, a resort near Santa Cruz, for the holidays. There were thirty of us total and each family rented a two bedroom condo on the bluffs overlooking the ocean. For Christmas Eve and Christmas Day dinners, we crowded into one unit and set out folding tables and chairs in a long row to accommodate all of us. It was noisy and boisterous but Perry had always been in the thick of it, giggling, his face red and his body jiggling with laughter. He always made a point to connect with each niece and nephew, even the most reticent and shy ones. He organized outings, kayaking in Elkhorn Slough, a movie in Santa Cruz, or a bonfire on the beach while I spent hours at the mahjong table with my mom and sisters.

This year would be the first time many of them had seen Perry since his brain injury and the admonition from the occupational therapist hung in my mind. "Don't put him among large crowds and make sure he doesn't get over-stimulated," she had said. I had considered canceling earlier in the week because I didn't feel strong enough to face everyone and didn't want to be the object of pity. Besides, I had to work right up to the 23rd because I had used all my vacation days during Perry's hospitalization, but my sister Rosemary persuaded me to come.

"I won't be able to help you make artichoke dip and deviled eggs and get everything ready," I told her. "Plus I don't know how Perry is going to handle being in such a large crowd. I don't even know if I can handle Christmas." We had not traveled out of town with him or been on any long car rides with him since his discharge from Casa Colina.

"Just come," she said. "It won't be the same without you."

Christmas Eve dinner was usually filled with loud conversation and laughter but this year, as we walked into the condo, there was silence. A somber hush filled the room and I wished we hadn't come. *Just treat me normal*, I wanted to say to all of them. All thirty of them—my mother, sisters, brother, aunt, their spouses, nieces and nephews—lined up near the door in a receiving line, looking at us with sadness and tears as they hugged Paul, then Zack, then me and Perry. I moved through the line, greeting everyone in whispered tones as we made our way to the long table. I helped Perry into his chair and sat down next to him as everyone took their seat.

Philip, my brother-in-law, stood and bowed his head to say grace. We were not a religious family but this was the one time, at Christmas, that we all united in a prayer to offer thanks. Philip always delivered grace because he and my sister Donna were the only ones that attended church.

In his heavy Chinese accent, he began, "Dear God, we gather today to give our thanks for all the food on this Christmas Eve and thank you for gathering the family and all their kids. We thank you for bringing everyone here safe from their long drives. We send a prayer to remember those who are no longer with us, Grandma and Jimmy [our stepfather] and we miss them." His voice quivered and broke. "We give thanks for Perry, that he is alive and able to be with us today. We pray that he will have more recovery. In the name of the Lord, Jesus Christ. Amen."

Tears ran down my checks. This was too sad. We should have just stayed in Los Angeles. I looked up and saw that my three sisters were crying, as well as many of my nephews and nieces. My mother looked down at her hands.

Philip surveyed the room, then clapped his hands. "Okay, let's eat," he said in an upbeat voice. Conversation started up again as people began to line up at the counter to fill their plates with our traditional menu: turkey, oyster sauce gravy, baked potatoes, chow mein, broccoli, corn and white rice.

Edward, our oldest nephew at age 33, sat to the right of Perry. He reached over and held Perry's hand.

"Hi Uncle Perry, do you remember me?" he said. Perry looked at him with a spark of recognition and his face broke into a grin.

"Edward!" he said, squeezing his hand in return.

"I'm happy to see you Uncle Perry."

"I'm happy to see you," he said.

Edward continued to hold Perry's hand while wiping his own tears with a Kleenex.

"Here, Perry, you don't have to get up," said my aunt Georgina as she handed him a filled plate.

Laughter and conversation filled the room again as the noise level got louder and louder. I worried that Perry would get distracted but he picked up his fork and ate with no problem. He was almost finished when I detected that faraway look in his eye, signaling that an agitation episode was imminent. I panicked. I needed to get him out of there. Maybe it was the noise, maybe it was too many people. We stood up and I walked him toward the door.

"What's wrong?" asked Rosemary.

"I think he needs to rest," I said.

Back in our own condo, I sat Perry on the couch and he leaned back, then closed his eyes. What was his tolerance for crowds and noise and what did this mean for family gatherings?

Was it now my responsibility to babysit him forever? Maybe this had been a bad idea.

There was a knock on the door. It was Dave, my aunt's husband.

"Do you need some help with Perry? Do you want me to help you bring him back?" he asked.

"No, I think it's too overwhelming for him," I said. "I think he needs to rest."

"I'll stay with Perry so you can go back and have dessert and visit with the family," he said. "Take as long as you like. I'll just sit here and watch TV with him."

I was flushed with gratitude when I went back to the family gathering. "Here, Auntie Cyn, sit here," said my niece Kellie, clearing a place on the couch. Rosemary handed me a slice of chocolate cheesecake.

When it was time to open presents, Zack escorted Perry back. It was as if he had just woken up from a long sleep. His eyes were clear and he was lucid. He smiled at everyone as we guided him to the couch next to me. After we opened presents, Rosemary sat on the other side of him. They had always loved bantering and teasing each other before his brain injury.

"Make a face like me, Perry."

Perry puckered his eyebrows and bared his teeth, looking fierce. I laughed along with my sisters and my mom as they watched.

"Make a face like Cyn."

Perry turned the corners of his mouth into a broad smile then looked at me. My heart melted. He was handling the large group just fine.

IN A QUIET MOMENT ALONE with my mother, she sat next to me and said, "I know the pain that you are going through. I have lived through all kinds of pain, too. I know what it feels like, a thousand needles jabbing you at one time. You will get through this."

Her words soothed me. We were united in our shared

tragedy, the loss of husbands, of lives cut short abruptly. I felt more connected to my mother than I ever had before.

"I know how tired you are, how hard it feels to face each day. I know what it feels like. But you need to take care of yourself. You are shouldering so much responsibility. Just remember to take care of yourself first because you can't help others if you don't," she continued.

I understood so many things about my mother in that moment. I had spent so much of my life not wanting to be like her but now I understood. What seemed selfish to me as a child I now saw as her drive for self-preservation, for assuring that her needs were met first. I understood her neediness, her desire to stockpile groceries, to have everything in place, so that in times of crisis when the world seemed scary and unknown, there would be this semblance of order. Her cupboards, her pantry, her house, her children were the only things that she could control.

"You need to stay strong for Perry and for Zack and Paul," said my mother.

"Yes, I know," I said. She didn't realize that she had been preparing me for this role since I was seven.

THE NEXT DAY PERRY AND I walked along the flat trail that circled the grounds of the resort on the bluffs. I was too scared to try the steep hike down to the beach, afraid he would lose his balance or that I wouldn't be able to get him to walk back up the trail. We stayed on the bluffs and at the lookout point, we leaned against the chain-linked fence, admiring the ocean below. "Does this look familiar to you, Perry?" I asked.

"Yes," he said, gazing at the ocean. "We've been here before." Then he turned to me. "It's all working out. You didn't think it would but it did."

I smiled and reached toward him to kiss his cheek. It was a nice Christmas present.

FOR CHRISTMAS DINNER, MY BROTHER always cooked a prime

rib. He would start fussing with the roast at noon, trimming the fat, adding garlic slivers and a hint of rosemary. That night the crowd had thinned to twenty but we still crowded around the folding tables and chairs. Perry had just finished his slice of beef when he stood up and turned to me, "I have to go to the bathroom."

I took him to the bathroom off one of the bedrooms but nothing happened. He stood up, walked into the bedroom, sat on the bed, then pulled down his pants. "Oh no," I groaned, "we just had a lovely day, not this." What do I do with my family out there and him in full blown agitation? "Please don't do this, Perry, not here," I said. He didn't seem to understand, he was already lost to me with that distant look in his eye. I pulled his pants up and led him out the door, through the living room and out to our own condo. Amid the noise of the family dinner, no one seemed to notice.

Back in our own condo, I let his restlessness take over. He pulled off his clothes, then put them back on. He took them off again and climbed into the shower. I turned on the water. He tilted his chin under the spray, letting the water wash over his face. Afterwards, I helped him dress but he pulled his pants off again and lay on the bed. I sat back, helpless. Was this how it was going be for the rest of our lives? Me sitting with Perry while my family parties in another room?

There was a knock on the door. I pulled Perry's pants up and walked him into the living room. Nick, our nephew and Mina, his girlfriend, were leaving.

"Goodbye Uncle Perry," said Nick. "It was really good to see you and you look great."

"Goodbye Nick," he said, as he reached to shake Nick's hand, then moved toward him for a hug. "It s nice seeing you."

The visit lifted Perry from his agitation. He sat on the couch again, calm, his eyes clear. A few minutes later, the boys returned with six of their cousins to play cards, followed by Dave.

"Hey Dad, let's play poker," said Zack.

"They're setting up mahjong" said Dave. "Go play. We'll be here to watch over Perry."

When I went back to the other condo, my sister Jeanne was emptying the tiles onto the green woven surface of the mahjong table. I hesitated. Would Perry be okay in the other room?

"Oh good, you're back," said Rosemary, pulling out a chair. "We're just picking our seats, it's a dollar a point this round."

I sat as we each drew a tile with a wind direction, east, west, north or south. My mom drew east and looked at the four chairs around the table, then picked her seat. "This one will be lucky tonight," she said as we arranged ourselves according to the direction on our tiles. In quick motions, we turned all the tiles face down then began the shuffle, the loud clattering of the plastic tiles and the jingles of my mom's bracelets competing with the TV in the background. Our fingernails jabbed each other as we moved the tiles in circular motions. I forgot about Perry in the other room as I listened to Rosemary dishing out gossip about old family friends. I stacked the tiles to make a row of eighteen, three in each hand to make six in a double row, just like my mother had taught me. It was a familiar and comforting motion and I felt my old self returning.

My mom threw out the dice after we finished building our walls of tiles then counted counter-clockwise. We retrieved our tiles in stacks of four, then opened them to arrange in a neat row. Before I could study my cards, Rosemary was already tapping her fingernails on the table. "Go! Take your turn!"

I smiled, thinking of all the years we had played together since we were young girls. I reached for a tile and studied what the others had thrown before I discarded. I felt my competitive spirit returning. My mother had taught me to not go for quick wins that paid fifty cents or a dollar, like my sisters. She taught me to study tiles and wait for the high point combinations or perfect hands that would yield $16 or $32 for a win.

I pumped my fists in triumph as my sisters cursed me in

Chinese each time I turned over my tiles in a big win. "*Thlay ngui*, how come you get all the good cards?" Rosemary said after I set my tiles face up in another win. My mom laughed as she counted my points, then reached in her money drawer. "She gets good cards but she knows how to play them, too." I giggled, happy to be with my sisters and mom again, happy that this part of my life had not changed.

When I went back to our condo that night, Perry was already asleep in bed. I changed into my pajamas and slipped in beside him, listening to his soft snores and the faint sound of waves crashing on the beach below the bluffs. This much remained the same, my family, my heritage. Not all was lost.

CHAPTER 17

—⁄⁄—

The week after Christmas, Uncle Ralph came for a visit. Perry had just finished his lunch and was sitting at the dining table with his eyes closed, his head swaying from side to side. Although he had greeted Ralph with a smile, he was sluggish and didn't initiate any further conversation. Ralph took a seat next to Perry and gazed at him with watery eyes.

"Gee, I was hoping for more progress than this," Ralph said.

Oh no, there he goes again, I thought. "Well, Ralph, we try to look at the positive, at what's come back," I said.

"It's just so tragic. He was so young, so full of vitality." Ralph's eyes filled with tears as he looked at his hands, mottled with age spots. He looked older than his eighty-two years. "I mean, he was such a successful lawyer and now this ...." He gestured toward Perry.

I sighed with impatience. I didn't need him telling me how tragic this was. He wasn't even related by blood; he married Perry's Aunt Molley and they never had children. Although they lived in the same city, Perry did not have a close relationship with them as a child. It was only after Perry graduated from law school and joined a big Los Angeles firm, that we were suddenly worth knowing and invitations to dinners, charity benefits, and concerts poured in. After Molley's death, the invitations continued and Ralph relished introducing us as "my nephew, the attorney, and his wife, the PhD."

"You have to let go of the old Perry; this is the new Perry," I said, trying to control the quiver in my voice. "You can look at the glass as half empty or half full," I continued. "We choose to look at it as half full and we are grateful for all the parts that have returned."

"Well, that's admirable that you can do that," Ralph said, shaking his head. "I can't."

Of course he couldn't. He could not conceive of a life with disability. Because Perry could no longer practice law in a prestigious firm or engage in witty conversation, he would be of no value to Ralph. Perry's ability to understand and follow conversations meant nothing. Did Ralph expect me to give up, put Perry in a nursing home, and walk away? Maybe Ralph was capable of doing that but I wasn't.

"Having him here in this condition is better than the alternative," I said, in a voice that was rising as my cheeks flushed with anger. "At least he is alive."

Ralph shook his head. "I don't know. If it was me, I wouldn't want this." He looked back at Perry who had opened his eyes and was following the conversation. "I don't consider this being alive."

I stared at Ralph, hating the way his large ears protruded from his head and his mouth that seemed too large for his face. I hated his tailored zipped jacket and collared shirt. I hated his neatly pressed khakis and shiny loafers. *If it was you*, I thought, *there would be nobody to take care of you because you disliked children and were glad you never had any. What do you know about the joys of being a father? You never had to give anything of yourself. What do you know about being alive? Your world consists of stock portfolios, investments, and donations to charity so you can see your name in print. You don't see Perry during his lucid moments, you don't see the spark in his eyes when he smiles at me or the boys.*

"He has the capacity to experience joy and love," I said. "He has the capacity to love his family still." My voice was getting shrill and I could feel the heat in my cheeks.

"Well, you can look at it that way. Me, I don't know if this is a life worth living."

I don't remember what else Ralph said during that visit. I just remembered wanting to yell, "*Screw you, Ralph. Get the hell out of my house!*" as he retreated down the front steps.

But the truth is that Ralph's words haunted me. Doubts began to creep in as the depths of Perry's deficits became more apparent. Did I really believe my own words about hope and optimism or was it false bravado? What makes a life worth living? I looked at Perry, sitting at the table with his eyes closed. Was he truly conscious? Was he aware of his surroundings? I had to believe he was, otherwise, why would I stay with him? Some evenings after a long day at work, I had to coax him to eat his dinner, scooping the food onto his fork, guiding his hand to his mouth. I wondered if it even mattered that I was the one helping him; would he fare just as well with any caregiver? The burdens on my life would be eased if I put him in a nursing home, but who would care for him with the same level of compassion and tenderness as me and the boys?

Without the ability to communicate and interact with others, to be aware of your surroundings, to experience emotions, and to draw on memories, what remains? When Perry was dazed and unresponsive to my questions, I felt foolish carrying on one-sided conversations. I missed our lively exchanges about our workday and what the boys were doing. He didn't remember what he did an hour ago or the day before. But still, I had to believe that he was in there somewhere, that I was reaching him.

ONE SATURDAY NOT LONG AFTER Ralph's visit, as I grew impatient during Perry's morning routine, I thought, *Maybe I have a bit of Ralph in me.* After Perry's shower, I toweled him off as he stood in front of the bathroom sink. I reached to lather his face with shaving cream but he turned away suddenly and I missed his cheek, smearing the side of his ear instead. I sighed, wiped his ear, then lathered again and handed him the razor. He placed it on the counter and looked into the mirror, expressionless. I picked up the razor and shaved his face, then trimmed his moustache, irritated by his mute silence.

"Talk to me, Perry," I pleaded with him. "Say something to me."

He slowly turned his face towards me, then smiled. His eyes became clear and alive, the vacant stare gone. He leaned in close to my face and grabbed my hands.

"Thank you for all the things you do for me," he whispered.

CHAPTER 18

─⊱✦⊰─

We established a new pattern in our lives with Perry home. On weekends, we went on walks at the jetty along the main channel in Marina del Rey, where all the boats headed out to the ocean. We rediscovered our favorite hike to Inspiration Point at Will Rogers Park in Santa Monica. We traveled east of downtown to visit the Huntington Gardens in San Marino or to Exposition Park to visit the California Science Center and the Museum of Natural History, all places we had always been too busy to visit. Paul and I felt the responsibility for keeping Perry engaged and stimulated at all times.

I wondered how much of our former lives we could reclaim. For the past ten years, we had shared season tickets to the Dodgers with a group of Perry's law firm partners. When the boys were younger, we attended each of our allotted six games. As the years progressed, our schedules grew fuller with other activities and we ended up giving away many of our tickets. This year we had the tickets again and I wondered if Perry could take on a Dodger game. Although it had been months since he had an episode of agitated behavior, I still had vivid images of what he was like at the height of his confused state. There were too many potential sources of worry in going to the game. How would we get him to his seat at Dodger Stadium? Once there, what would we do if he became agitated? Maybe it was just easier to stay home and keep him away from challenging environments.

"No, let's try it anyway," Paul said. "If he spaces out, we can just leave. Our parking is really close and we can leave anytime we want."

I reconsidered. The easiest thing to do would be to stay home and let disability limit our lives. But I thought about Dodger dogs, the peanut vendors and the chocolate malt ice cream I loved. We could face whatever challenges were out there. After all, Paul and I weren't brain injured, we needed to resume our normal lives with or without Perry.

One evening in April, Perry was sluggish when I got home from work. He was sprawled on the couch with his eyes closed and his hands clenched into fists.

"Come on, Perry, get your shoes on," I said, pulling him into a sitting position. "We're going to the Dodger game!"

He sat up, opened his eyes then he closed them again. He had always loved the Dodgers. Why wasn't he more excited? I reached to pull socks over his toes. Beads of perspiration formed on my forehead as I tried to shove his feet into his shoes. I was getting no cooperation from him.

Paul tugged on his arm. "Come on, Dad. Stand up."

Perry moved his weight forward but then sat back on the couch and closed his eyes. His shoes still dangled from his feet. I was about to give up and say forget it when Paul used a shoehorn and managed to get his shoes on, then helped him into his jacket and placed a Dodger cap on his head. We were going to that Dodger game, whether Perry liked it or not.

We guided him into the car and headed east on the freeway. We drove the familiar route downtown, then crawled slowly up Elysian Park Boulevard and pulled into parking lot 4. We could hear the roar of the crowd as we got out of the car. It was already the bottom of the first inning. Perry was now fully awake as we maneuvered through the crowd to aisle 100. At the top of aisle, I paused, facing the long flight of stairs down to our seats in row G. Were those steps always so narrow and was the pitch always this steep? Even when the boys were five and seven, I didn't worry about them falling down these steps. But now I worried about Perry's uneven balance.

Paul went down the steps first so that he would be able to break his fall in case he lost his balance. Next went Perry, holding firmly onto the handrail. I trailed behind, my hands hovering near his waist in case he faltered. Slowly, we made our way down the steps to row G.

Once settled in our seats just to the right of home plate and above right field, I looked around the stadium. Chavez Ravine glowed in the setting sun and the Elysian hills and San Gabriel Mountains had a purplish hue. The crowd cheered when the Dodgers got a base hit and I looked at Perry, who was smiling as he watched the game. He caught my eye and his face was lit with a wide grin. It was as if a switch had been turned on inside of him. As the next Dodger scored a base hit, he cheered along with the crowd.

When Paul brought us Dodger dogs and garlic fries, I worried that Perry would become distracted and I would have to feed him. But he ate without assistance while keeping his eye on the game. When he finished eating, I cleared away the wrappers and napkins. He began squirming in his seat, making motions to get up from his seat.

"What's wrong?" I asked, nervous that he wanted to leave. He slowly raised himself into a standing position and I was poised, ready to help him if he decided to make his way to the aisle. As the roar of the crowed passed over us, Perry raised his arms in unison with the group around us. "Yay!" he cried. In my vigilance over his well being, I missed the "wave" of cheering fans that washed over our section.

I sat back and let out a sigh. He was more aware of his surroundings than I was. For the past six months, I avoided large gatherings, afraid of how he would respond. In time, I would learn that, in contrast to the literature on brain injury, Perry was more stimulated in challenging environments. At home, in his carefully controlled, quiet world, he grew sluggish and passive. He thrived with more stimulation.

Whenever the Dodgers scored a run, Perry stood with the crowd. "Wooo!" he would say, a decibel higher than his normal voice but not loud enough to be considered a yell. At the seventh inning stretch, we stood, waiting for the organ to play the opening stanzas. "Take me out to the ball game ..." sang Perry, as he swayed with the music. "Root, root, root for the Dodgers ...."

At the bottom of the seventh inning, I turned to Perry. "Do you want to stay for the whole game?"

In the past, he would usher us out at the top of the eighth inning, or the bottom of the eighth, if he was generous.

"Aw Dad, do we have to?" the boys would protest. "Can't we stay till the end of the game?"

"No, if we get out now," Perry would say, "we'll beat the traffic. Besides, I have to get up and go to work tomorrow morning." If it was a weeknight, Perry would add, "Plus, it's way past your bedtime." The boys would reluctantly gather their belongings and we would listen to Vin Scully broadcast the rest of the game on the way home.

This time, Perry turned to me and said, "Yes, let's stay for the whole game."

We watched the Dodgers beat the Expos, 13-4. Baseball had returned to our lives.

Chapter 19

— ⋋⋌ —

I dabbed holy oil onto my index finger from the small brown vial then rubbed it on Perry's forehead. He looked at me with his eyebrows arched, curious. Smiling back at him, I recited the prayer on the back of the laminated card in my broken Spanish:

"*Dios, infinitamente santo y glorificado enmedio de tus santos, Tu que inspiraste al santo monje y ermitano Charbel para que viviese y muriese en perfecta union con Jesus Cristo, dandole la fuerza para renunciar al mundo y hacer triunfar desde su ermita, el heroismo de sus virtudes monasticas: pobreza, obediencia y santidad.*"

God, infinitely holy and glorified among your saints, You who inspired the holy monk and recluse Charbel to live and die in perfect union with Jesus Christ, giving him the strength to renounce the world and to triumph from his seclusion, and rewarded him with sainthood for his monastic virtues of poverty, and obedience.

IT WAS APRIL 2004 AND the holy oil and prayer were gifts from Nancy who had just returned from a visit to Mexico City. Her host, Tomas, was a descendant of the family of Saint Charbel, a Lebanese monk known for his healing miracles.

"I told him about Perry's heart attack and brain injury," said Nancy. "Every time we visited a church, we lit a candle and said a prayer for him. On our last night in Mexico City, Tomas gave me this holy oil and said to rub it on Perry's forehead, then say the prayer."

I took the vial and studied the laminated card with the picture of Saint Charbel, his weathered face, white beard, and the black angelic cowl. On the other side was the prayer printed in Spanish.

"I don't know if you even believe in this," said Nancy. "But maybe you can try it?"

Nancy was accepting of alternative healers and psychics, but she knew I was strongly grounded in western medicine and skeptical of new age and unconventional remedies.

"Of course I will try it," I assured her. How could I refuse a gift that was given with love and sincerity?

Saint Charbel lived a monastic life with a Maronite order in Lebanon. He took a vow of poverty and obedience then devoted himself to manual labor and piety to God. He spent 23 years in silence, living as a hermit. He died in 1898 at the age of seventy and, after his burial, a series of miracles appeared. A great light emanated from his grave. When his body was exhumed four months later, it was intact and oozed a blood-like moisture. No one could explain why his body had not deteriorated. A nun with severe intestinal problems prayed at his grave site and was cured. Almost a hundred years later, in 1996, oak leaves blessed by Saint Charbel healed a woman who had lost the ability to walk. Could this vial of holy oil blessed by Saint Charbel perform miracles on Perry also?

Although I didn't believe in miracles, what did I have to lose? I had reached the end of the road with western medicine. After three months, our health insurance stopped paying for speech, occupational, and physical therapy. I knew that close cadre of support working in harmony had been too good to be true. Our family doctor wrote a letter to our health insurance advocating for more treatment to no avail. She wrote a referral to a neurologist in the hopes that his assessment would carry more weight.

When that coveted referral finally came, I was excited when we met with the neurologist. But he was indifferent and cold when I asked him about neuropsychological testing and another MRI. "What's the use?" he had said. "Look, nothing is going to make him any better." And before I could ask him about alternative treatments like hyperbaric oxygen or neurofeedback, he was already halfway out the door. "It's too bad," he had mumbled, shaking his head. "I'm sorry."

The reality of Perry's condition was there in black and white, neatly typed in the discharge summaries from the rehabilitation center. Each phrase cleaved deeply into my heart. Each phrase delivered a cold, stark piece of reality.

"He has poor initiation with notable poverty of content," read the discharge summary. "He will continue to experience difficulty with confusion and orientation, difficulty with concentration, poor memory and recall for recent experiences, fatigue, and irritability." I remembered the speech therapist at the rehabilitation center explaining to me, "He doesn't initiate speech and when he does speak, it's always in response to your question, usually just one word or two. He doesn't respond to his environment or what is happening to him."

And then there was the monthly progress report and the single phrase written by the speech therapist that signaled the end of insurance coverage. He wrote that "…a leveling off trend has been established in most treatment modalities," and it was the justification the insurance company needed to halt further therapy sessions.

The medical community had given up on Perry and written him off. But I didn't believe their words and couldn't accept it. How could I continue to hope for improvement? To admit that he "will experience permanent impairment in functional ability" was to admit defeat. Why not rub holy oil onto his temple and forehead and pray?

"*Te imploramos nos concedas la gracia de amarte y servirte siguiendo su ejemplo.*

"*Dios todopoderoso, Tu que has manifestado el poder de la intersection de San Charbel a traves de sus numerosos milagros y favores, concedenos la gracia (…) que te imploramos por su intercession. Amen*"

We implore you to grant us the grace to love you and serve you following his example.

God almighty, You who have manifested the power of intervention in Saint Charbel through his numerous miracles and blessings, grant us the grace for (…); we implore you to intercede on his behalf. Amen.

I WONDERED IF PERRY COULD hear the desperation in my voice as I recited the prayer, could sense the force of my touch willing him to get better as I dabbed his forehead with holy oil. I wanted to believe in the power of prayer. I wanted to believe that the strength of my love would heal him, that I would be able to reach into the damaged neurons and synapses in his brain and repair them with my touch.

Was I not pious enough? Did I need to undergo some type of penance in order for him to get better? Saint Charbel spent the last 23 years of his life in solitude, leading a life of purity, obedience, and self-deprivation. Did I need to devote more of my life to Perry's healing? I was now his case manager without the cadre of support from the medical community. I devoted myself to the holy oil, anointing Perry every night and faithfully reciting the prayer. I wasn't ready to give up yet. I had to believe he would continue to improve.

To my amazement, he did. Each day, each week, it seemed as if he woke up a little bit more, as if he was improving. Or was I just seeing the intensity of my desire for him to get better? Still, it seemed, he woke with a little more alertness each morning, a little more clear-eyed. His long periods of staring off into space, drooling, oblivious to his surroundings faded. He looked at us straight in the eye when we asked him questions. When he first got home, he would give me a blank stare when I asked what he wanted for dinner. We scribbled questions on an erasable whiteboard, "Do you want pasta or chicken for dinner?" and drew in boxes for "yes" and "no" for his response. He would take the marker in his hand and limply check the box. But now he answered us right away.

Perry's face lit up with a brilliant smile, full of delight and surprise whenever he caught a glimpse of me. Instead of seeing a man with severe cognitive deficits, I saw the man I loved pre-brain injury who used to call me several times a day just to hear my voice, the man who arranged a private car for me when I visited New York alone on a business trip, the man who, for my birthday, searched used bookstores in the entire city of Los Angeles to find the next mystery book in the Swedish series I was reading. His brown eyes sparkled when he laughed at our jokes. He thumb-wrestled with the boys and played punching games with Manny. On walks, he clutched my hand tightly, switching hands around his back when we changed sides so he didn't have to let go of me.

ONE SATURDAY AFTERNOON IN MAY, I scanned the newspaper for events. "Don't let him sit around and watch TV all day," the occupational therapist admonished me. "That's the worst thing to do for brain injury patients. He needs stimulation." *A movie on a big screen*, I thought; *that should fill up the afternoon.* We could walk around the mall after the movie. I dragged Perry into the car. He was sleepy when I pulled into the parking structure; his eyes were closed, his head leaning forward. When I walked to the passenger side to help him out of the car, he refused to move.

"Come on, Perry, the movie is starting," I said.

He shook his head side to side and didn't move, his eyes still closed.

"Don't you want to see a movie?" I asked.

He shook his head again, no.

"Come on, get out of the car."

I pulled on his hands, tried to swivel his legs outside of the car. He pulled his legs back in.

"No," he said, opening his eyes and looking at me, defiant. "I don't want to see a movie."

I couldn't wedge his 160 pounds out of the front seat of the car. Frustrated, I gave up and drove home. I threw the keys on the kitchen table, angry that a simple task could reduce me to tears. How was I going to get him to improve if he wouldn't cooperate? The weight of responsibility for his healing, for keeping him stimulated, felt insurmountable.

I steered Perry into the backyard and parked him in a lounge chair in the shade, then surveyed our landscaping. Our garden was in desperate need of weeding. The year before, we had put in new plants. Now, a year later, the new shrubs and fruit trees were beginning to fill in. The camellias were blooming; the plum tree was flowering. The side yard between the garage and our neighbor's fence was lined with bamboo on one side, and deep pink cannas on the other. Gray flagstone pavers created a path to the back of the garage, surrounded by mossy baby's tears. But now weeds sprouted among the patches of bare dirt, and throughout the baby's tears in between the pavers. I squatted down to pull out the sprouting crabgrass weeds. I could feel my anger and frustration dissipating as a cool breeze rustled through the bamboo plants. I inhaled the smell of the rich, brown earth. I had forgotten how peaceful and comforting a simple task like weeding could be. Before Perry's brain injury, I loved to garden, loved the smell of the earth and the sense of accomplishment I felt when I saw our well-tended plants. I forgot about movies and malls and brain injury as I pulled weeds, one by one.

When I stood up again, the bed of baby's tears looked pristine again. Drake sniffed the ground near me. A lone bird chirped in the distance and I could hear the faint tinkle of chimes from our neighbor's backyard. Perry dozed in the lounge chair, head tilted forward.

What was so wrong about having unstructured moments like this? His refusal to get out of the car was an improvement. He showed initiation in telling me what he didn't want to do. He conveyed his own desires and was aware of his environment. Did I really need to fill our weekends with frenzied activity? In my quest for events to spur on his healing, I had not stopped long enough to consider how my life had changed. Did his healing necessitate a life of self-deprivation for me? How was I going to find meaning and fulfillment? What I really needed to do was take care of myself and my own healing process.

Months later, I had lunch with Manny. I had been dabbing the holy oil and reciting the prayer religiously each night.

"You seem to be at peace with this. I notice a new sense of serenity and calmness about you," he said.

"Really?" I didn't feel any different. My sorrow was always there, lurking in the background.

"Yes, I notice a difference in you. You seem more accepting of this all."

I suppose I was more accepting of Perry's condition. Each day, each month, I saw small improvements as more of his essence returned. In the clinician's eyes, he would never be whole again but he was complete enough for me. I didn't spend my weekends rushing from one activity to the next and I didn't worry about keeping his brain constantly stimulated. We spent hours on the couch watching TV if we wanted or read magazines in the backyard. I wasn't paralyzed by sadness anymore; I didn't wallow in sorrow; and I wasn't in a constant state of anger. I had learned to carve out time for moments of solitude, for writing and reflection.

"You know, the person that gave Nancy the holy oil said it may or may not have a direct effect on the person with the brain damage," Manny continued. "He said maybe the miracle will be on those who surround him."

It wasn't until I received the English translation to the prayer that I realized the "(...)" in the prayer meant I was supposed to recite Perry's name. In all those months of faithfully reciting the prayer in my broken Spanish, I never inserted anyone's name.

Chapter 20

~\|/~

A year after Perry's heart attack and brain injury, I received a promotion at work to a director position with increased responsibilities and now supervised a staff of 35. I moved from a cubicle into a private office where I could speak openly with Perry's therapists without worrying about my colleagues eavesdropping. I was mastering a whole new set of skills in terms of managing employees, delegating tasks, and directing workflow. My workdays were full but I felt in control, content almost, buoyant with resilience.

But I worried about Perry and how he would make meaning of his new life. I thought about his attorney days, which were filled and overflowing. He left the house at seven in the morning and often came home after seven in the evening, after the children had been fed and bathed. Some days he didn't have time for lunch and ate a candy bar from the vending machine. He had looked forward to an early retirement and wanted to transition out of his busy attorney life at age fifty to make whirligigs in the garage and putter around the house. He was retired now, in a sense, but incapable of making whirligigs or puttering in the garage. The caregiver took him out to lunch and on walks in the neighborhood or the beach. I continued physical and occupational therapy once a week without help from insurance but it wasn't enough to fill his days. I thought he needed more activity to fill in those empty blocks on his calendar. I didn't want him to sit in front of the TV day after day.

I found a day-treatment center for brain-injured adults in Torrance and exchanged a flurry of excited phone calls with the director as she told me about their program. The goal was to help members regain independent learning skills. It sounded ideal for Perry. But when we visited, the room was a cold, cavernous warehouse with concrete floors and fluorescent lighting. The members sat around four round tables, listless and quiet, eyes glazed from medication. It reminded me of my volunteer days in Santa Barbara at a center for mentally ill patients. I remembered the colorless walls, the impersonal rooms and the sense of boredom and monotony among the patients. I shuddered. I could not reconcile my image of the old Perry with the one that would be sitting at the game table, vacantly staring at a card game. Even in his diminished capacity, I couldn't picture him there.

I visited a newly built senior center with his physical therapist in Culver City. We peered into yoga and aerobics classes, "oohed" and "ahhed" at the glittering swimming pool, and admired the polished exercise machines. I felt hopeful as we walked to the social worker's office through hallways with blonde wood flooring, sunlight streaming from high windows. But then the social worker said she was sorry, Perry didn't qualify to use the facility because he wasn't aged fifty or older. Besides, they didn't offer any classes or activities for brain-injured adults.

Then I found the Acquired Brain Injury Program at Santa Monica College. Sandi, the director, was effusive and enthusiastic on the phone. The program had a variety of classes geared to all levels of brain injury. There was a weekly "Connections" class where participants went on community outings to museums, enjoyed picnics at the park or the beach, attended brain-stimulation classes, and did problem-solving exercises.

"Come to the assessment class," Sandi told me. "It's the first step and then we can determine what is best for your husband."

The assessment class was in a classroom setting with seven other students working silently on a questionnaire while the instructor sat behind a desk at the front of the room. I had thought he would be given a one-on-one assessment but each person was to fill out the questionnaire on their own. I leaned forward to read the first paragraph. The assessment class was geared toward finding his current abilities, interests, and goals, it said. My stomach tightened as I looked over the next six pages. There were open-ended questions about the nature and course of his brain injury, therapy treatments, physical health, social/emotional status, cognition, memory, communication, and academic background. The instructor wanted each student to fill out the questionnaire without assistance but I knew that the severity of his brain injury would make this task too challenging for him. Maybe this assessment class was a big mistake.

Although he could read and comprehend the questions, his handwriting was tiny and microscopic, a condition called micrographia where he scribbled small, cramped words. His previously sloppy handwriting was now even more illegible. He also had a tendency to perseverate, where he repeated the same action over and over until he was told to stop. When given a pen to write, he would start by writing normal-size letters then drift into smaller and smaller letters. He then repeated circles and loops until the page was filled with ink spots. He was not going to be able to write legible, short answers on this questionnaire on his own.

Perry had already picked up the pen and was writing microscopic letters after the goals.

"Wait," I said. "Give me the pen."

I moved to the sections with open-ended questions and

drew two boxes under each question and labeled them "yes" or "no." I pushed the questionnaire and pen back to him and told him to check off the boxes. He methodically worked through the document, checking off the "yes" and "no" boxes. When he got to the question, "Do you have memory problems?" he checked "no."

I sighed. He was unaware of his deficits. Even though I had told him repeatedly what had happened to him, he was always surprised. The information never got lodged into his long-term memory so he never acknowledged there was anything wrong with him. There was a medical term for it—"anosognosia"—where one is unaware of his or her deficits due to brain injury. Maybe it was better this way—that he was unaware of the depths of his brain injury to spare him the profound sorrow we all felt.

I wondered what the administrators of the program would be able to distill from his answers on this questionnaire, especially if he wasn't even aware of his deficits. I hoped that this assessment class wasn't an exercise in futility and wouldn't be like all the other places I had visited that turned out to be inappropriate for Perry. If it happened again here, what would I do? What other options did I have?

I looked out the classroom window at the sky gray with fog and at the branches of the eucalyptus trees rustling in the light breeze. At two in the afternoon, Santa Monica was still swathed in foggy June gloom. *I can't do this.* I felt the urge to bolt from my chair and run into the grayness and disappear, away from the confines of the classroom with Perry and his caregiver sitting patiently, away from this life of responsibility and brain injury.

Instead, I turned back to Perry and watched as he checked "no" to "Do you have difficulty remembering events that occurred or persons you knew before your injury?" and "Do you have problems concentrating?" Then he came to the question, "Do you use memory aids?"

He checked "yes," then proceeded to write in microscopic

letters next to "What types of memory aids?"

"Wait," I said. "What are you writing? Do you use memory aids?"

"Yes," he said, as he looked up at me and paused in his writing.

"What memory aids? What do you use?" I asked.

His eyebrows were knitted in concentration as he pointed to the microscopic letters he had just written with his pen. "My wife."

Sandi called me a week later. "I don't think the 'Connections' class is the right place for him at this time," she said.

I knew it, I thought, as I felt a sting of tears in my eyes. I had gotten used to hearing "no." I was trying to hide the disappointment in my voice and thinking of how I could end this call when Sandi added, "But there is a computer class that I think would help with his language skills. We also have a speech-communication class in the morning on the same day so he can do both—the speech class in the morning, have a break for lunch, and then the computer class. There's also a physical fitness class for stroke victims that meets two days a week. I know he didn't have a stroke but they focus on stretching and conditioning and I think it would be good for him."

It took a moment for that to sink in before I felt my shoulders loosening, my tension eased. "That sounds wonderful!" I said, my face breaking into a smile.

In the following weeks, the empty blocks on his calendar began to fill up with classes as I entered them into an organizer. One Saturday, we were at the grocery store when an older, gray haired woman came up to us.

"Hi Perry, how are you?"

I didn't know who she was. I looked at Perry to see if he recognized her. He smiled as if she was familiar and said, "Hi, it's nice to see you."

"I'm in your class at Santa Monica College," she said, then

turned to introduce herself to me. "I see him every week at exercise class. He doesn't talk much but it's good to see him out and about!"

I smiled back in return, grateful that he had found a life independent from me and that he was part of a new community.

CHAPTER 21

—√⁄—

It is his voice that I miss so much, that deep, resonant voice that sprang from within and carried, that made the boys jump to attention when it was sharp. "Speak from your diaphragm," Perry used to tell me. "Your voice is so soft, it doesn't carry. My mom always told me to speak from my diaphragm." Then he would take a deep breath and sing out, "THEN EVERYONE CAN HEAR YOU." Now, after his brain injury, that voice elicited brief bursts of euphoria when I heard it, unpredictable, fleeting, and ephemeral.

We discovered that if you gave him a phone, he used his normal voice, rather than his usual hushed whispers. It puzzled us but we used it to our advantage. If he didn't respond to a question, we called him on the phone, even if we were in the same room. But his conversations did not always follow logic.

One day, I called home from work and Perry answered the phone. I had forgotten to tell the caregiver to drive the silver car today because Paul needed the green car after school.

"Hello?" he answered in a loud and clear voice.

My heart skipped a beat. *It's back! His voice is back!* "Hi Perry! Have you had breakfast yet?" I asked, happy to hear his normal voice.

"I don't know … I think so."

It was 10:00 in the morning. Most likely he had already had breakfast but didn't remember.

"Perry, I need to talk to Norman. Can you give him the phone?"

"Who?"

"Norman, he's the guy who is helping you today."

"Norman? There's nobody here by that name."

Of course he wouldn't remember Norman by name; he was the replacement caregiver that day. Our regular caregiver, Leonard was out for the week. Most of the times he remembered Leonard by name since he had been with us for six months.

"Yes, there is. He's the Filipino gentleman that is helping you today. His name is Norman. Can you call him to the phone?"

I tapped my pencil on my desk with impatience. While I was delighted to hear Perry's voice, I had things to do and needed him to surrender the phone to the caregiver.

I heard him put the phone down on and say softly, "Norman, phone. Pick up the phone, Norman."

Of course Norman couldn't hear him. I could barely hear Perry. He must not be in the same room. He picked up the phone again.

"No, there's no Norman here," Perry said, in his normal voice into the telephone.

"Perry, there are only two people in the house right now, you and Norman. Can you please get him to come to the phone?"

In the background I heard beeping from the microwave oven. Norman must be in kitchen.

"I think he's in the kitchen, Perry. Can you stand up, go in the kitchen and hand him the phone?"

"No," he said.

"Why?"

"I don't know what he looks like."

I sighed in exasperation. I had learned to take the good and the bad of his condition. While it was wonderful to hear his voice again and this encounter was good for a chuckle, the reality was you couldn't hold a decent conversation with him.

THAT AUGUST, ON A SATURDAY evening, Perry was lying on the couch after a day of dazed silence. I knelt beside him. "I hope you have a better day tomorrow," I said.

"Me too," he said as he cupped my head with his hands. He looked at me with lively eyes, full of love.

I studied his face, every freckle, every wrinkle, the scar on his forehead when he ran into a wall as a child, the way his eyebrows arched perfectly and the thin lips hidden by his moustache. I knew this face so well, as I've watched it change from adolescence to adulthood to middle age. This face was so familiar to me, yet could seem so foreign when one of his eyes wandered to the side and the faraway brain injured look appeared.

"You were kind of spacey and tired today," I said.

He nodded in agreement. I studied those freckles again, the ones near his right earlobe that still had a solid pebble-like hole from his piercing. I liked to rub the lobe and feel that little bump, a reminder of what he once was and what hasn't left him.

"I hope you will talk more tomorrow," I said. "I wish you would talk to me more, like you used to."

He mumbled. "I wish you could fi … me."

I leaned in closer. "What did you say? Fight me? Find me?"

"You have to find me," he said in a clearer voice.

My heart beat faster. "Are you in there somewhere?" I asked, my voice rising.

"Yes."

"Do you want me to find someone to help you with your speech?"

He nodded his head more vigorously. "Yes."

If Perry had stopped speaking entirely and never uttered

another sound, I would have agreed with the health insurance company and given up hope. If he spoke consistently, we would have known the true extent of his cognition, and I would know what to advocate for. But it was the unpredictable and variable nature of his responses that spurred me on and fueled my hope that he was truly there. The random and haphazard times that he spoke with clarity and lucidity kept me going, kept me from not giving up and continually searching for resources to help him.

I knew that the rehabilitation therapists viewed me with skepticism or thought I was delusional when I insisted that parts of his cognition remained and that he remembered facts from his life as an attorney. Although he was often silent and spaced-out during evaluation sessions, at home with me, he often answered in a clear and audible voice.

"What's a docket?" I asked.

"It's a calendar for court hearings," he answered.

"What's twenty-seven plus thirty-four?" I asked when I was filling out tax forms and too lazy to reach for the calculator.

He replied, without hesitation, "Sixty-one."

I learned to read his gestures, his eyes, his smiles. They conveyed the connections that were no longer carried by speech. I could sense when he was there, when his eyes were lively, darting around the room, alert to movement and his surroundings, when he smiled and his cheeks took on a rosy glow, when a glimpse of his former self emerged. But just as quickly, it would turn. He would close his eyes and shake his head from side to side. When he opened his eyes, I could tell he was gone, the liveliness faded, the vacant stare apparent again.

I devised strategies to get him to respond. I prompted him to signal thumbs up or thumbs down. I typed questions on the computer, and in more lucid moments, he typed coherent responses.

"Perry, why are you so quiet today?" I typed.

He typed back. "I can be loud or quiet today. Which do you want?"

"I would like you to be talkative."

"Ok I'll do it," he typed, but he whispered for the rest of the day.

I NEEDED TO FIND A speech therapist who would believe that the essence of him remained and that he was worth working with. I followed leads from rehabilitation hospitals, friends, and searched websites in Los Angeles until I found Geri. She seemed intrigued by his case, and in the first session she focused on him intently, questioning, observing, and patiently waiting for his responses.

"It's all in there still, filed away in different cabinets in his mind. We just have to find the right key," she said. There were no vocal chord exercises. "We need to create webs of information for him. It's like a spider web; all the information is in there, but we need to create those connections for him."

The long-term memories were what he remembered best and could respond to, Geri told us. We typed questions to orient him: the ages of the boys, where he went to school, where he practiced law. One of his problems was initiating speech. She taught us to help by starting answers for him. Once he got started talking, it was easier for him to continue. So when we asked, "What do you want for breakfast?" we prompted him with, "Say, I want ..." and he would reply, "I want cereal."

One weekend we circled the aisles at the grocery store, looking for lunch choices.

"Do you want sushi or a sandwich for lunch?"

He gave me a blank stare.

"Do you want sushi?" I repeated. "Say ... yes or no."

Again, the blank stare.

"Do you want a sandwich?" I paused, waiting for a response. "Say ... yes or no."

His face broke into a smile and a mischievous glint in his eye appeared.

"Yes or no," he said.

CHAPTER 22

⛤

I longed to get back to the wilderness. During our camping trips pre-brain injury, it was the one place where Perry truly relaxed, away from the pressures of work. I loved him most in that environment, fishing pole in his hand, worry lines erased from his face. We spent our days hiking and fishing or perched on granite boulders, reading.

Perry had introduced me to backpacking the summer after our freshman year in college on an easy four mile hike through a densely wooded forest to Grant Lake in the western Sierras. We were caught by an afternoon thunderstorm and while lightning struck trees around us and thunder rumbled through the valley, torrential rain pelted us. I shivered in my wide bell bottom jeans, inappropriate for the wilderness and my fake hiking boots called "wafflestompers" that I bought at a discount store. My long, polished nails broke when I tried to pound in stakes for the tent and unravel knots in the rain fly. We unfurled our sleeping bags once the tent was up and waited out the storm in Perry's orange two-man tent, hugging each other to keep warm.

I fell in love with the wilderness on that trip, mesmerized

by the smell of the earth, pine needles and hint of juniper. I had never seen such deep blue skies, such clear water. I was never aware that such serenity and natural beauty existed in the world. Through the years, I became more experienced in the wilderness. I walked with confidence when the Vibram soles of my Pivetta hiking boots gripped the granite surfaces when we boulder hopped. I knew how to keep myself hydrated and warm, recognized the signs of altitude sickness, learned how to read the curving lines on topographic maps and could find carats to direct us to the proper trail. When we had children, we resumed our wilderness trips by having horses carry our gear. The boys learned to love the wilderness as much as we did and the highlight of our summer was our trip to the Sierras.

Perry's heart attack and brain injury had put a stop to any thoughts about camping. He was no longer able to hike long distances and I could not imagine helping him into a sleeping bag at night, fumbling with zippers and flashlights. But still, I longed for a glimpse of the wilderness, even a day hike into the mountains to feel the wind on my face and hear the sound of a stream rushing over rocks.

That summer, a year after his heart attack, we planned a five-day vacation in a condo at Mammoth Lakes in the eastern Sierras. There would be no horse packing or camping out but we planned a variety of day hikes to get into the mountains. The first morning, we filled our day packs with water bottles, sandwiches and snacks, then boarded the shuttle bus to the trailhead for Rainbow Falls. We had planned on hiking three miles roundtrip to Rainbow Falls, then taking the bus to Devil's Postpile. At home in Los Angeles, Perry had hiked two miles in the local mountains with no problem.

As we got off the shuttle bus at the trailhead, the driver said, "You should take the loop trail to Devil's Postpile." He had heard us talking about the hike. "It's only about a mile longer and it's level. If you come back to this trailhead from Rainbow Falls, you have to go uphill."

A mile longer would mean a total trip of four miles. Paul,

Zack and I looked at each other and shrugged.

"Sounds good to me," I said. Maybe it was the thin mountain air or the grandeur of the Minarets, but my mind didn't register the true distance. It was twice as long as any distance Perry had hiked since his heart attack.

Perry walked with ease on the gradual downhill trail in the pine forest, his steps slow but steady. I inhaled the familiar scent of juniper and pine, exhilarated. Halfway to Rainbow Falls, the pine forest gave way to a devastated burn area from a wildfire in 1992. The terrain was dotted with broken stumps, bare pine trunks and decaying logs. We squinted in the bright sun but Perry made it to Rainbow Falls without becoming winded or tired by the time we stopped for lunch. On a bench at the overlook, we peered down to the falls, where the San Joaquin River spilled 100 vertical feet into a pool. Hikers scampered over rocks to frolic and swim in the pools at the base of the falls but the hike down seemed too strenuous for Perry. He seemed happy and relaxed on the bench, looking at the falls.

We ate our sandwiches and refreshed, we headed for the loop trail to Devil's Postpile. We didn't realize that the trail cut through another burn area. Instead of a shaded trail, we hiked along a dusty path in the hot July sun. Bare poles of pine trees, stripped of bark and branches, rose from the barren landscape resembling a tree ghost yard. Puffs of dirt and sand rose with each step in the soft gravel and pumice, coating the inside of our nostrils. After a half mile, Perry began to lag, due to the heat, the dust, and the high altitude. We stopped to rest but there were few rocks or logs to sit on and no trees for shade.

The boys had walked ahead of us but as Perry and I fell further behind, they circled back to join us. I made Perry drink water each time we stopped. Then he began to pitch and sway as if he was going to lose his balance. Paul rushed to grab his right side while I held on to the left. We walked together for a few yards, then Perry stopped again and looked at me, his eyes tired and unfocused.

"Are you okay, Perry?" I asked.

He nodded yes. We had another two miles to go. I questioned my sanity in bringing a brain injured man into the wilderness. How could we have thought four miles was no big deal?

"It's okay, Dad, we'll just take it slow," said Paul.

But as we slowly inched along the trail, Perry stopped walking. We looked for a place to sit. There was only a wide rock, low to the ground. Perry sank onto the rock and looked like he wanted to lie down. We let him rest so he could regain his strength. Five minutes went by, then another ten. I held the water bottle to Perry's lips to get him to drink. What if we couldn't get him to stand up? I worried that we would have to summon paramedics in here to carry him out.

"Come on, Perry," I said. "Get up, let's keep moving."

He shut his eyes and didn't move.

"Come on Dad, it's just a little further and then we'll hit the shuttle bus. Can you stand up?" asked Zack.

Perry remained seated with his eyes closed.

A man with graying hair in his 50s hiked past us, alarmed, "Do you need help?" he asked.

"No," I waved him on. "We'll be okay."

I was too embarrassed to ask for help. I hadn't thought about consulting a doctor before we came to Mammoth to see if there were any precautions we should have heeded, bringing Perry to high altitudes. If we had to, the three of us would carry him out of there. As I sat on the rock with Perry in the direct sun, dust coating my clothes, face and hair, flies buzzing around us, I was filled with despair. The prospect of a future without the wilderness was unbearable. *Don't take this away from me, too.*

Another five minutes passed then Perry opened his eyes and let us help him stand, supported by Zack and Paul. We began the slow shuffle step walk toward Devil's Postpile, stopping every 50 yards to let him rest. I didn't pay much attention when we reached the basalt columns. I was focused on getting him on the shuttle bus, less than a quarter mile away. When we climbed aboard and sat on the hard bench seats, that quarter mile seemed like ten miles. I looked at Perry. He flashed me a wide victory smile and slept very soundly that night.

TWO DAYS LATER, REFRESHED FROM the hike, we drove to Mosquito Flat, the trailhead for Little Lakes Valley in Rock Creek. Skittish about taking Perry on another long hike, we decided that Mosquito Flat would take us closest to the high Sierra since the trailhead was at 10,300 feet. Near the parking lot, I studied the map. Mack Lake was only a half mile up the trail. Maybe he would be able to hike that far?

"We could always just turn around if he stops walking," said Zack. We headed up the path, skirting the gushing creek up the canyon. A profusion of red Indian paintbrushes, pink columbines and deep purple lupines lined the trail. Perry walked behind me, cheery and with his fists clenched, holding his arms out for balance and not clutching me. Paul followed behind Perry, ready to catch or steady him in case he stumbled. My spirits lightened when we crested a hill and Bear Creek Spire, Pyramid Peak and the grandeur of the valley came into view. We hiked off the trail and settled on rocks overlooking Mack Lake, the water a deep aquamarine blue amid the granite peaks.

I looked at Perry, sitting on the grass, leaning back on a rock eating a plum. He caught my eye and smiled. He had the same air of serenity he always did when we came into the wilderness. Zack and I took out our books and read while Paul and Perry dozed in the warm sun, savoring the thin mountain air and the sound of the waves on the lake lapping on the shore.

ON OUR WAY HOME TO Los Angeles, we saw the sign for the Ancient Bristlecone Pine Forest. Perry and I had brought Zack there when he was four months old but we weren't bold enough to try a hike with an infant and didn't see much of the park.

"Let's check it out," said Zack. "We're in no rush to get home."

We turned east from Highway 395 and climbed 25 miles up to the White Mountains. I would have been happy to just tour the visitor's center but Zack wanted to hike the loop tour of Schulman Grove to get closer to the trees, the oldest living things on earth. I was still nervous about hiking with Perry, afraid that he would stop walking again.

"But it's only a mile," said Zack. "He did fine yesterday."

We set off on the one mile loop trail. Perry walked with no problem and needed no support from any of us. He kept a steady pace and smiled in admiration of the thousand year old gnarled trees twisted into bizarre shapes. Benches lined the trail so there were plenty of places to stop and rest.

It was a new experience for us all, visiting a place that none of us had seen before. At the end of the trail, we ate lunch on a picnic table in the shade. I marveled at the resiliency of the trees, how they continued to grow for thousands of years in spite of the alkaline soil and barren landscape. I studied our family sitting at the picnic table, Paul fiddling with his camera, Zack resting his feet on the bench. Would I succumb like all the other plant life in the area, unable to live in this bleak environment? Or was I going to be like those trees, twisted and bent, learning to adapt and thrive under the harshest of conditions?

CHAPTER 23

─◖◗─

In January of 2005, Paul left home to spend a semester of his junior year in high school at the High Mountain Institute (HMI), located outside of Leadville, Colorado. The school offered a high school curriculum in the wilderness where students learned Science, English Literature, History and Math while they backpacked on expeditions. Months earlier, when Paul told me he wanted to apply, my initial response was "No! No way!" I couldn't handle caregiving by myself. I needed his help with Perry, with meals and all the chores around the house. Since Zack had left for college, it was Paul who would see my exasperated sighs or tears of frustration and tell me it would be okay. It was Paul who would offer to take care of Perry when I was at my breaking point, ready to scream. I already missed Zack's presence and help. I couldn't imagine how I would cope without Paul.

But I could see in Paul's eyes the hope for escape and freedom from the burden of caregiving. He had this responsibility thrust on him while his friends worried about driver's licenses and SAT's. He was sullen and sad most of the time. There were evenings when he answered my questions with mono-syllabic responses, then closed the door to his room.

What had happened to my little boy who was all sweetness and light? He was born with blonde hair, which darkened with age. He resembled Perry with his light coloring and sprinkling of freckles and I often wondered where the Chinese side of him went. As a toddler, he loved his "monkey-dance" where he would hop from side to side, kicking out his legs while tapping his belly and laughing. He said, "Thank-you, Mom!" whenever I served him Eggo waffles or nachos for snacks. He was at my elbow in the kitchen while I cooked, asking questions and helping me grate cheese. When I quit working to stay at home with the boys, Paul and I spend leisurely mornings together after dropping Zack off at school. I pushed his stroller up the hill to the community gardens. We walked among the dirt paths admiring the blooms of sweet peas, sunflowers, cauliflower and broccoli. Paul would run ahead, then point to me with wonderment, in his soft, lilting voice, "Look Mom! A broccoli! A zucchini!"

I longed for that Paul again. Now I saw frown lines and glum adolescence tinged with sorrow. He withdrew more socially. Apart from a few close friends, no one at his school knew what he was going through with Perry. He took on more responsibilities at home when he got his driver's license; he grocery shopped, picked up pet food for the dog, got take-out dinners or cooked before I got home from work. He didn't ask for material things, he wasn't interested in cars or clothes. The best gift I could give him was freedom, escape from caregiving and disability.

I turned to Paul. "Yes, you should apply. It would be a wonderful opportunity."

THE NIGHT BEFORE PAUL LEFT for HMI, he filled up both cars with gas, then went to the drug store and bought five packs of Depends diapers. "I know how it's a hassle for you," he said.

The next morning, I dropped him off at the airport and watched as he hoisted his heavy backpack from the trunk and onto his shoulders. He turned back to give me a smile. He seemed to have grown even taller than his current six-foot frame in the last few days.

"Don't worry about me, Mom, I'll be fine," he said.

I held onto him for a moment longer than usual, tears welling in my eyes. "I'll miss you."

"I'll see you in a couple of months when you and Dad come to Colorado. You are going to be fine, Mom. Plus, you always have Manny and Nancy across the street," he said. I watched until he disappeared into the double doors and headed for the line to check his baggage.

I got on the freeway and headed downtown, inching along in rush hour traffic. We had raised our boys to be independent and adventurous yet at that moment, I wished I had insisted that Zack defer college or go to a school in Los Angeles, or that Paul not go to HMI. In spite of my bravado in front of Zack and Paul, I was terrified. There had always been someone with me while I was caring for Perry, another person to sympathize with, to call on for help. I worried about whether I would be able to handle Perry on my own. I wondered if I would turn into a raving lunatic because I didn't have anyone else there to help me.

At work, I was occupied in meetings all day, then Perry and I went out to dinner with friends. It wasn't until we returned home later that evening that I noticed the heavy silence in the house. Only the jingle of Drake's dog tags and his eager trot greeted us. Always, there had been the background noise of a sports program on TV, or the throbbing bass of music from the boys' room, or the clacking of keys on the computer keyboard from the den. The silence was unnatural, sobering. My heart lurched when I walked by Paul's room and saw his empty bed, books and magazines still strewn on the floor. I missed seeing his notebook on the kitchen table, the ice hockey gear in the doorway.

As the weeks passed though, I began to feel a sense of

serenity when I returned and found books and magazines on the coffee table exactly the way I had left them. There were no crumpled towels on the floor in the bathroom, no empty containers of Gatorade on the end tables. For dinner, we could eat a salad or nachos or a sandwich without having to worry about cooking a complete meal with a protein, starch and vegetable. Paul was always hungry. When he was home, I cooked hearty breakfasts on the weekends, with bacon, potatoes and eggs. An hour later, he would ask, "What's for lunch?"

During his weekly check-in calls home, I could hear Paul's happy, jolly self returning. He was loving HMI and was full of stories about the new friends he had made, their wilderness expeditions and the leadership skills he was learning at the institute. He was relieved that I hadn't collapsed in heap of discontent over him being gone.

I found that Perry was easier to handle on my own. Somehow, having one less person to worry about or plan meals for made my load seem lighter. There was no one to get mad at for not taking out the garbage cans or forgetting to feed the dog or picking up the dog poo. There was no feeling that the other person was not pulling his weight, there was only me. Even Perry seemed more calm, more cheerful, when it was just the two of us.

One Saturday afternoon, I settled onto the couch and rifled through the channels with the remote control. When Paul was home he always watched his favorite sports shows. I pressed buttons on the remote control and switched it to "All Channels." I was surprised. We had access to many more channels than ESPN and other sports channels. I could watch Oxygen or the HG Network or TLC.

"What do you think, Perry? What do you want to watch?"

He turned to me and smiled. "Whatever you want. I'm happy with whatever you want."

I leaned back into the sofa. I thought of how many times I had given in to the demands of children, my husband, my mother, without thinking of what I wanted. In our previous life, I always deferred to Perry to plan the next vacation, choose the restaurant for dinner, decide where to invest our finances. Although I considered myself independent and "liberated" as a female, I depended on him to make decisions, to take control. He was resolute, determined while I tended to waffle in making decisions. Now, I was free to make choices based on my own needs and wants, rather than the needs of others. I could take control rather than feel that it was being imposed on me, I could dictate the path.

IN APRIL, PAUL WANTED US to come to HMI for Parent's Day. I wanted to see it, too, based on all the stories he was telling me about the main lodge and its spacious kitchen, the yurt where they held classes and the log cabins that they slept in. I wanted to meet his teachers and his new friends.

But I had never traveled with Perry, just by myself. I always had either Zack or Paul or both when we flew on an airplane. They were able to accompany Perry to the restroom when we couldn't find a unisex or family bathroom, help with the luggage, and jump in if Perry became unstable or agitated. The reality was that in another year, Paul would be going off to college. I didn't expect Paul to stay close to home and I wanted him to expand his horizons, like Zack did by going to NYU. I was going to have to face the prospect of traveling on my own.

Could I do it? In the three months that Paul had been gone, handling Perry by myself turned out to be easy. His agitation episodes had long faded. He accompanied me to the grocery store, to the mall, and he sat patiently while I got my hair cut. So what was so hard about getting on an airplane to Denver with him and driving two hours to Leadville? The worst that could happen would be that he would soil himself and I wouldn't be able to find a bathroom. But was that enough to keep me from visiting Paul and seeing what HMI was like? I decided to forge ahead.

I was nervous when the caregiver dropped us off at the airport. We went through security lines with no problem but as I was paying for magazines at the airport newsstand, I noticed Perry grimacing. He usually did that when he had to go to the bathroom. As I got closer to him, I could smell that he had soiled himself. I looked up and down the concourse. There were no unisex or family bathrooms at LAX. How was I going to get him changed? Although every public restroom had a disabled symbol indicating they had handicapped stalls, they were either located in the women's room or the men's room. I didn't feel emboldened enough to walk him into either.

Then I noticed two security guards standing idle at a booth. I walked up to them, leading Perry by the hand. They looked up and smiled as I approached.

"Hi, I need help," I said. "My husband is disabled and needs assistance in the restroom. Are there any unisex or handicapped restrooms I can take him into?"

The first one scratched his chin. "Hmm, I don't think so. Not in this terminal. There are handicapped stalls in the restrooms."

"I know, but you have to walk into the men's or women's rooms."

He nodded in understanding. The second security guard stood up.

"Come with me," he said. "I have an idea."

He started for the stairs to go down to the lower floor. "There's a restroom down there that gets very little traffic. I'll stand outside and guard it so that no one comes in while you help him. The only bad thing is that you will have to go through security again."

That seemed like a small price to pay for privacy. "No problem," I said.

He led us down the stairs and stood in front of the entrance of the men's room. As I helped Perry change in the stall, I heard the guard telling people, "Sorry, this restroom is temporarily closed right now."

Afterwards, I thanked him profusely as we walked back to the lines to go through security again. *There.* The worst thing I imagined happened but we got through it. Another hurdle was passed.

IN DENVER, WE STAYED AT the Brown Palace, splurging for a night of luxury amid the mahogany walls and ornate grillwork, before heading to the mountains. Perry was groggy in the thin air but I stayed up late watching TV and listening to the faint strains of the piano in the atrium lobby through our door.

The next morning we climbed to 10,000 feet as we drove into the Rockies to reach Leadville. I felt competent and accomplished—I had done it on my own and had not hit any major snags so far. At HMI, we toured the cabins, I met Paul's teachers, we sampled the delicious food prepared by students. The thin air and high altitude was hard for many of the parents and several needed supplemental oxygen, but we did fine. Even better, I didn't sense a hint of awkwardness over Perry's disability; he was embraced and welcomed by students and parents alike.

At the end of the weekend, Paul flew home with us for spring break. The flight home seemed even easier with his help. After buckling Perry into his seat belt, I leaned back in my seat on the plane and smiled. I had done it. I had traveled with Perry by myself.

CHAPTER 24

⁓⋇⁓

After spring break, when Paul had returned to HMI, I heard water running in the pipes in the middle of the night, filling the toilet, then stopping. That didn't sound right. In our previous life, I would have nudged Perry awake.

"Perry, there's something wrong with the toilet."

And he would say, "What? When?" and sit up, throw off the covers and get out of bed, go into the bathroom. He'd lift the cover the tank, stare at it, jiggle the handle and know what was wrong. It would necessitate a trip to B and B Hardware in the morning, then maybe another trip because the part he got would be too wide or too narrow but eventually the right part would be found and the toilet would run water only when we flushed and remain silent all other times.

Perry had loved crawling under the house to reconnect phone lines or untangle speaker wires. He examined latches on gates, washers on leaky faucets and connections on electrical wiring. No challenge was too great for him. But now, after his brain injury, he wasn't capable of diagnosing the toilet or fixing it, either. He stared at me when I asked him why we would hear water running in the toilet.

"I don't know," he said.

In the morning, I lifted the cover of the tank, peered inside. I never fixed a toilet before. What was I supposed to find?

I led Perry into the bathroom. "Does anything look broken to you? Do you know why water is running in the toilet?"

"No," he answered, shrugging his shoulders, peering into the tank. "I don't know."

I browsed through *Dare to Repair* by Julie Sussman and Stephanie Glaskas-Tenet but got lost at the diagrams of angle adaptors and overfill tubes. I called Manny and he came over from across the street.

After looking at the tank, he said, "You need a new fill valve. See? The stopper is corroded so it's leaking water and the tank fills when the water gets too low. We need to turn off the water to the toilet, then remove the piece."

He showed me the knob at the base of the toilet to turn off the water and then took out the faulty valve.

"I can replace this for you. Do you want me to go to the hardware store?"

I considered his offer. It would have been easier to say yes and have him do it for me. But I needed to learn this; I didn't want to rely on a man to get things done.

I put the part in a plastic bag and went to B and B Hardware with Perry in tow. It used to be his favorite place, a small neighborhood hardware store with narrow aisles crammed with merchandise, floor to ceiling. This was not a place to push a shopping cart and browse. We found the plumbing section with toilet repair parts and I scanned the wall. Every nook and cranny of the aisle was filled with some kind of part related to toilet repair but none of the parts matched exactly what I had in the plastic bag. I picked up one toilet valve set that kind of looked like the one in my bag and handed it to Perry.

"What do you think? Would this part work?"

Did the brain injury erase all that knowledge about home repair or would this toilet valve spark a neuron that would bring it back? I remembered reading an article by a woman in an automobile accident and suffered traumatic brain injury. Before her accident, she was an accomplished cook. After her brain injury, her friends came to teach her how to cook again and she reported that each ingredient and measuring cup felt like a foreign object to her. She had to relearn everything.

I wondered if the same thing was happening in Perry's brain, if all these hardware parts were foreign objects to him, with no meaning, no purpose since he lost so much of his memory. He reached for the valve part and turned the package over.

"I don't know," he said.

I stood bewildered, then found a salesman to help. He took the part from my plastic bag and searched through the rows of displays.

"This one should work," he said. "We don't have the exact same one, but this valve is the right size and it should do the job. If not, you can always bring it back."

I sighed. So that's why it always took several trips to the hardware store whenever Perry did repairs. Only this time it meant I would have to get him in and out of the car again, hold his arm while he walked slowly to the store and down the crowded aisles with me. I was really hoping this valve would work as I buckled him into his seat belt in the car.

We stopped at the grocery store on our way home and as I was backing out of the parking space, I waited for a middle-aged couple to pass. They looked a few years older than us, the wife with short gray hair in jeans and a sweatshirt, the husband with thinning hair, khaki pants, tennis shoes and a sweater. A gust of wind came up while they were walking and he stopped, then reached to zip up his sweater. I took a deep breath. The cool air felt sharp in my lungs. My chest tightened with longing. "How wonderful," I thought, "to have a husband who can zip up his own sweater."

Back home, I took my book and new parts into the bathroom, ready to install the valve. I had to read through the instructions in *Dare to Repair* several times. Although the book was geared toward women with no knowledge of home repair and written in clear understandable language, my eyes glazed over when I read about the shank washer, cone washer, O-ring, coupling nut, and angle adapter.

Why hadn't I paid closer attention when Perry was trying to teach me how to fix a leak in the bathroom faucet? He explained how washers worked and gaskets, but I was only half listening. I had stood in the doorway, my book in one hand and watched as he twisted and turned the faucet to show me the washer and gasket. I yawned and said, "Can I finish reading my book now?"

I turned the knob at the base of the toilet to turn off the water, then went outside and turned off the water main leading into the house just in case. I remembered all the times Perry did plumbing jobs and cursed when water came gushing out of a faucet or pipe. I spread a towel on the floor and looked at the parts. Following the instructions, I put in the new valve with one hand and fit the locknut on the supply tube with an adjustable wrench in my other hand. I connected the refill tube to the angle adapter and clipped it to the edge of the overfill tube. Then I went outside to turn on the water main, and back to the bathroom to the knob at the bottom of the toilet to open the water flow. I stood back and flushed. Then I waited. The tank filled to one inch below the overfill tube and stopped. I waited for another minute. The toilet remained silent. I raised my fist and pumped my arm. Success!

CHAPTER 25

—ᵥᴵᵥ—

I had always loved road trips. Starting with the four hour drive from Salinas to Santa Barbara during my college days, the open road symbolized freedom, adventure and the prospect of something new. After college, Perry and I drove to the Midwest to become VISTA volunteers and I loved the carefree feeling as we drove away from classes and obligations, all of our possessions packed in the back of his Datsun pick-up. After we had kids, we loved long driving vacations with the minivan filled with snacks and games for the boys.

But that summer, when Zack was home, I wasn't too excited about our road trip to Leadville, Colorado to pick up Paul from HMI. The week before our departure, Drake had stopped eating. It took several days for the vet to diagnose a mass in his abdomen that was too big to operate. We waited for a few days more, hoping for a better prognosis but finally agreed with the vet that it was best to put him to sleep.

I packed with a heavy heart. Reminders of Drake were everywhere, his water bowl still on the floor, his container of dog food and his leash on the counter. I wouldn't ever hear the jingle of his dog tags again, the rumble when he burst through the dog door, his scratching at the gate, his loud lapping of water from his bowl, his jumping up and down as I filled his bowl with food.

I packed duffle bags in haste with clothes and whatever snack foods we had in the house. I worried if I had anticipated all that Perry would need: Depends, bed pads, shower bench, medications, extra clothes. I worried about how he would fare being in a different motel room every night or whether he would find the road trip disorienting. He had a set schedule every day and responded well to the structured activities of therapy and exercise classes.

As we drove east, the open road was soothing and helped keep my sadness at bay. By the time we passed the neon lights of Las Vegas and then the orange sandstone cliffs and verdant farms in Utah, my mood lightened. I felt my worries lifting as we sang to the Beatles and Rolling Stones, Perry singing along with me.

Zack provided entertaining diversions. He made up games for us to play while we drove, like "Jingo." The first person to spot an American flag or an overly patriotic display of red, white and blue scored a point when they yelled, "Jingo!" He was filled with an adventurous spirit and childlike enthusiasm. I felt the same sense of fun and amusement like I did when the boys were young and we played endless rounds of "Guess What I'm Thinking," and "I Spy With My Little Eye," to keep them occupied and curious.

When we reached Ruby's Inn, near Bryce Canyon, I felt freer and lighter, something I hadn't felt since right after college. After we checked in, I browsed through our guide books. "Should we book all the other nights, too?" I asked Zack. "What if all the hotels are filled and we can't find a place for the night?"

"No, let's be spontaneous," he said. "Let's just play it by ear and see where we land every night."

I loved the idea of meandering. Pre-brain injury, I was always the one who wanted to linger or stray off the main path to explore when we traveled. But Perry's limited vacation days meant that every moment mattered, our schedule needed to be planned in advance, with a printed itinerary left with his secretary so he could be reached. Even when he was away, he was linked by phone, e-mail and fax. There was always some emergency that needed tending, some important case where his expertise was needed. So what was stopping us from being spontaneous now?

The next morning, we drove to Sunrise Point in Bryce. The carved cliffs and pinnacles were beckoning in their orange, pink and yellowish glow. We had visited this park twice before, once when Perry and I were in college and again when the boys were three and five. Both times, we weren't able to hike into the canyons because of deep snow. Now, in late May, the trails were clear. However, the guidebook did not recommend the strenuous hike on steep trails for visitors with health problems. I thought about Perry's difficulty with balance and decided we couldn't risk hiking into the canyons. We walked along the easier paths at the rim instead, Perry slowly stutter stepping while holding my hand. I gazed at the orange hoodoos lining the sandstone canyon, disappointed that another opportunity to hike into them was lost.

We left Bryce following Highway 12, where the ochre and orange rocks gave way to monochromatic rocks, striated in differing shades of gray, contrasted with the deep blue sky and vivid green hay fields. It was late afternoon by the time we headed north toward interstate 70 and Green River after visiting Capitol Reef National Park.

"Let's stop at Goblin Valley State Park," I said to Zack, while studying the map. "It's a little ways off the highway, but not too far."

As we headed off the main highway, I could hear Perry's voice from the past, grumbling, "It's too far away, it's already 5:00 in the afternoon, we'll be eating dinner late and we don't even have a place to stay for the night!" I tried to shake off the worry. That was how we traveled in the past. We were exploring new pathways now, being spontaneous and developing a different mode of travel, I told myself. Still, a little nagging doubt remained. What if something happened and we couldn't find a place to stay?

When we reached Goblin Valley, my doubts were erased as we gasped in surprise. The wind had carved the soft red sandstone into waist high formations of spires, gnomes, and goblin-like creatures. Even Perry looked amused as we spilled out of the car and onto the soft sandstone. Zack scurried to take photos in the setting sun while Perry and I wandered among the rock formations, following the well-worn trails. He touched the sandstone while he shuffle stepped on the trails and smiled when we topped another rise and saw more goblin-like stones. I wondered if this was what his everyday experience was like. His lack of short-term memory meant that every experience was new; at each stop, he was viewing it all with a sense of awe and discovery, as if he was seeing it for the first time. For a brief moment, I had that same feeling of delight.

THE MOST DIRECT ROUTE TO Leadville would have been to stay on Interstate 70. But the next morning, Zack studied the map.

"Let's try to hit as many national parks as we can," he said. "There's one called the Black Canyon on the Gunnison. We can go south and then drive up to Leadville." And so we headed toward Delta, past green fields and farms ringed by the snow covered Rockies. At Crawford, we turned off the highway and onto rural roads to reach the north rim. At the first overlook, we hiked to the edge of the deep canyon. My toes tingled and I felt a lurch in my stomach as I peered into the canyon, trying to capture the depth of the sheer vertical walls on my camera. In the past, I would have clutched Perry's hand because I was scared of heights but this time he squeezed mine. I guided him to the guard rail, worried that his shuffle step would make him lose his balance.

"Are you scared, Perry?" I asked.

He grabbed the rail, peered down, then looked up at me

with a wide smile. "Nooo," he said. "Are you?"

From our map, it looked like a road connected the north rim to the south rim. But there was no road, we would have to backtrack two hours to get to the main highway to continue south. I worried about Perry again; we should have had lunch an hour ago. There were no towns nearby and we had no snack food in the car. It was 3:00 in the afternoon by the time we stopped for lunch. Perry ate his sandwich in big gulps but there were no adverse effects. He seemed to be handling spontaneity just fine. Maybe I needed to lighten up, like Zack, taking each day as it comes, not worrying about routines or structured schedules.

THE NEXT MORNING, WE WERE united with a jubilant Paul in Leadville, bursting with stories of treks into the wilderness, pranks he and his classmates pulled on their instructors, tales of the bonds he had created with the students who had gathered at HMI from all parts of the country. After packing his gear in the van, we debated whether we should head south again through Utah or north to the Rockies. We had four days to make our way back to Los Angeles. None of us had been in the Rockies so we set off for the national park.

Just inside the entrance, we stopped at the first overlook and snapped a photo of the snow capped peaks under dark cloudy skies. Three miles later, when we stopped at the visitor center, rain began beating against the van. Undaunted, we pressed on, determined to drive the Trail Ridge Road through the park. The rangers assured us the road was open all the way to Estes Park in the east, even though the road reached elevations above 12,000 feet. As we progressed, it began to snow, and Trail Ridge Road was shrouded in fog.

I drove clutching the steering wheel, white knuckled, wishing Perry could drive. I hated driving in the snow and Perry always handled hairy driving conditions with his steady hand. I didn't trust the boy's driving enough to surrender the wheel as neither of them had experience driving in snow or ice.

We passed signs for the Alpine Visitor Center, Moraine Park, Beaver Ponds but all we could see were gray clouds and fog. My shoulders began to ache from gripping the steering wheel so tight and my eyes were strained as I crept along, keeping the Toyota in front of me in view, afraid that I would drive off a cliff without those tail lights guiding me.

The boys lapsed into a tense silence as snow and fog covered us with unease. Although I was happy to see Paul and loved hearing his stories, there was a shift in the mood in the car. Paul didn't share our sense of adventure, he didn't feel a part of our happy, spontaneous troika. He was longing for his buddies in his wilderness program. Zack got tired of his stories and Perry was silent. We spent the rest of the day in silence, shrouded in a gray funk.

We all felt a sense of relief when we dropped from the gray and cloudy mountains, back into the high desert outside Arches National Park. The next morning, everyone's mood brightened and the boys were up for an adventurous hike into Fiery Furnace, a maze of slots and arches. In the past, we would have gone into Fiery Furnace as a family, anxious to escape the touristy crowds on the easier hikes, happy to seek a sense of isolation in the wilderness. This time, I dropped the boys off at the trailhead then felt wistful as I drove to the Windows section of the park for an easier half-mile hike with Perry. We walked slowly to several arches on the flat trails. *This is not so bad*, I thought. I could still see arches, I could still enjoy national parks and the outdoors. After our hike, we drove back to Fiery Furnace to wait for the boys. I gave Perry an apple and bit into mine while I opened my book and settled in for the wait.

The boys arrived back at the car right on schedule. Then Perry began coughing. We patted his back and he spit up a piece of apple. His coughing subsided. He was breathing normally and his coloring was fine. Energized from their hike, the boys were eager to explore Canyonlands next. By the time we reached the north end of the park, Perry was coughing again, as if he had something lodged in his throat. I could hear him wheezing.

"Are you okay, Perry?" I asked.

He nodded yes.

"Are you having trouble breathing?"

He shook his head no. But he coughed and coughed then grew red. Alarmed, I stopped at a turnout and got him out of the car. Paul performed the Heimlich maneuver but nothing happened. It looked like he was having trouble breathing. Zack stood outside the car, watching.

"Let's take him to the hospital," said Paul.

We got back in the car and headed south toward Moab, in emergency mode, anxious, on the alert for a blue H hospital sign.

"There it is!" cried Paul and we headed down a residential street to a two story hospital. At the emergency room parking lot, Perry was still coughing, his face red, as I helped him out of the car. The waiting room was empty and by the time we got Perry seated on one of the plastic chairs in the lobby, he had stopped coughing. His normal coloring had returned. The triage nurse approached us.

"My husband choked on an apple and he's been coughing but we can't tell if he's okay because he had an anoxic brain injury and he doesn't initiate speech," I said in one long breath. The nurse's eyes widened. Without taking him into an examination room, she sat next to Perry and felt his neck.

"Can you breathe?" she asked Perry.

"Yes," said Perry, nonchalant and with his normal tone of voice.

She stood up and got a cup of water from the cooler nearby.

"Drink this," she said. "Let's see if you can swallow."

Perry picked up the cup and took a big gulp, swallowed with no problem, then smiled at her.

"I think he's fine," she said to me. "He obviously can swallow so there's no obstruction. If you are really worried, we can take an X-ray but I don't think it's necessary."

Relief washed over me. Since his heart attack, we took each

calamity seriously. We left the hospital and abandoned our plans to drive further south. We found a motel room in Moab and ordered take-out food since we were too tired to venture to a restaurant. The hospital episode was yet another reminder that we would be on a constant vigil over Perry's health.

As we drove south to Arizona the next day, spirits were glum. There was no time for extended hikes, no meandering off the interstate, no spontaneity. We only had two days left to get back to Los Angeles. This was what traveling with brain injury was really like.

"Our fun meter is dependent on how Dad's doing," said Zack, in the driver's seat, after we crossed the Arizona border.

"Yeah, I know," I said, thinking that we would forever be at the mercy of his abilities or lack of ability. I looked out the window, wondering how we could capture that feeling that we had at the beginning of the trip, the sense of fun, of excitement. I picked up the guidebook to find a place to spend our last night on the road.

"Let's pamper ourselves," I suggested. "Let's stop in Sedona, I've always wanted to visit that town."

It was twilight by the time we checked into our spacious two-room suite at the Enchantment Resort. The setting sun cast a peachy orange glow on the red rocks surrounding our room. We ordered a lavish room service meal, complete with appetizers, entrees and dessert. After dinner, we spread out on the two king-sized beds. The soft down comforter and sage scented pillows lulled me into a contented, satisfied silence. This trip was so much like Perry's path of recovery, with moments of happiness and carefree exuberance, then punctuated by worry over his health. That's the way our lives would be from now on.

But at least we tried, I thought. We got him out and on a road trip and saw as many national parks as we could during these five days. We didn't back down and didn't hide at home. We still had our sense of adventure and we were learning how to live with disability.

CHAPTER 26

~⟍⎪⁄~

Later that summer, I was standing at the refreshment table at Perry's "graduation" from his stroke support group, feeling content and happy with myself for having found this resource. Perry had attended the program for the last six months, sponsored by the American Stroke Association. Two days a week, the group offered sessions with occupational therapists, lectures from medical experts and social activities where he was encouraged to talk and sing. It had been a good setting for him.

Charlotte, whose father was in the stroke group, joined me at the refreshment table.

"This group has been so wonderful. There are no places like this, no doctor ever tells you about this," she said, her face terse and without a smile or trace of happiness. She placed her hand on my arm and I noticed her manicured, painted nails, a soft pink hue. "My father had his stroke four years ago and he was in Alaska, deep sea fishing, can you imagine?" she said.

She looked older than me, in her 50s, with dyed blonde hair in a pixie cut, striped knit top and twill pants. But her face was twisted into a permanent scowl that her heavy foundation and pastel lipstick could not hide.

"Yes, I can imagine," I said. "My husband had a heart attack while we were vacationing in Portland for a bar mitzvah."

"I dropped everything and flew up there," she continued, not acknowledging what I just said.

"You know, in Alaska, they have such hard lives that if you make it past 50, they consider you having lived a full life. After three days, the doctors wanted us to pull the plug, they had no hope. He was in a coma for six weeks. It was terrible and our lives changed overnight."

I nodded. Every person, every family in this room had gone through the same thing. "Yes, I know," I said, "you can't anticipate these things."

"It was a nightmare. I camped out in the hospital once we got him to Anchorage, then we had him medically evacuated back to Los Angeles. And then what were we supposed to do? What is there to do after that? None of the doctors even told us about these kinds of groups. Many of us didn't even know there were support groups for caregivers because we don't consider ourselves caregivers."

"I know," I said. I wanted to add that we had done the same thing, but Charlotte was not interested in hearing my story.

"No one tells you these things," she continued, her voice bitter as she took a sip of punch. "You have to find everything out on your own. My husband and I moved out of our home in the valley to live with my mom and dad in Bel Air. We have given our lives over to his caregiving."

I looked over at her father in his wheelchair. He was talking to one of the stroke group members with halting, slurred speech. *At least he can speak*, I thought. He looked well cared for in his polo shirt with a stiff collar and his tan Faconnable windbreaker. His silver hair was neatly combed and he was clean shaven. His wife hovered nearby, in a starched blue button-down shirt and pearls. Her face, like Charlotte's, was etched with worry. Unlike the smiling and laughing stroke group members surrounding her, she didn't break a smile.

"Don't you have a full-time caregiver?" I asked. They must have ample resources, judging by their appearance and their residence in Bel Air.

"Sure, but I have to help out with all his activities and doctor's visits. What else are we supposed to do? Who else is there to help? I have given up my life to help my dad." She folded her arms in a defensive pose, her face in a grimace.

I studied the creases in her forehead, the way her face rested in a scowl, her lips pressed tightly together and thought, *This is what I could have become. This is how I could have reacted. Bitter. No joy in the world.* I was relieved when Sheila, the wife of another stroke victim approached us. Her husband, Bob, was in the same exercise class with Perry at Santa Monica College.

"It's a Godsend, finding all these classes," said Sheila. "I see Perry all the time but I don't see you. Do you work?"

"Yes, I do. I work for the school district downtown."

"I used to work for the school district, too. I was a preschool director but I had to quit my job after Bob's stroke."

She looked away and I could sense the wistfulness in her voice.

"I was nearing 65 anyway and then this happened," said Sheila. "So I quit to take care of Bob. I could have kept working. I loved my job."

"I think that work saves me," I said. "When I am at work, my life feels normal and my mind is taken away from disability."

"Yes, you are lucky you can do that," she said. "But I feel like Bob needs me. Don't you feel that way about Perry?"

I paused. I remembered the days at Casa Colina when it seemed like he was more alert and aware when I was there. I often wondered if he would improve at a faster rate if I was with him. I remembered when one of Perry's law firm partners said, "You must feel guilty for working so much now that this has happened." But I didn't feel guilty. I liked working. Was I not as caring as Sheila?

As I drove into the office after the stroke meeting, I felt

unsettled. Was I doing the right thing by working so much? I was engaged and enthused about my work, even on those busy days when I didn't have time to sit at my desk or answer e-mails until the end of day. I liked being able to immerse myself in a world where my sole identity wasn't being the wife of a brain-injured husband.

I wondered what my life would be like if I tended to Perry full-time. His disability insurance was ample enough that I could afford to quit work. But what would be the shape of my life? I imagined the conversations with other caregivers, the discussions of therapies and medical procedures and the constant mourning over what was lost and what once was. I wasn't as noble as Sheila who gave up her career to tend to her husband. I imagined myself bitter and resentful like Charlotte as I shuttled Perry from one activity to another.

Ever since graduate school, I had deferred to Perry's career which had eclipsed mine in terms of salary and prestige. His job had always come first and I happily acquiesced. I was able to stay home with the boys when they were young and go back to school full-time for my doctorate. But when I went back to work, it was always me that made accommodations when they were sick or stayed home when the sitter couldn't come. When Perry traveled for work, our household didn't skip a beat but when I went on a business trip, I had to leave instructions and field endless phone calls on where the music lessons were or what time baseball practice ended. Now that I was assuming leadership at work, I didn't have to defer to his job anymore. Although I did take time off to arrange his therapies and activities, I didn't have to hold back at work. My job was demanding and frustrating at times but it was my escape into the world of normalcy. I was too selfish to give that up entirely.

CHAPTER 27

～ﾉﾉ~

Later that summer, during my annual physical exam, my doctor detected a suspicious mass on my ovary. Ultrasound revealed a small cluster, like grapes clinging to my left ovary as well as fibroids in my uterus. Surgery was the recommended option, although the doctors didn't feel it was life threatening and did not think the surgery needed to be scheduled immediately.

A tingle of alarm swept through me. *What if it's cancer? Not now! Not after everything we have been through with Perry! This isn't fair!* I thought about my mother who had just passed away from lung cancer the year before, even though she had never smoked. For a year, she went through rounds of chemotherapy but eventually succumbed to the cancer. If my case was serious, the doctors would have recommended surgery right away. But even if it wasn't cancer, I didn't know if I was ready to surrender my uterus and ovaries. At 49, I was nearing menopause and my child bearing years were over. Zack and Paul were entering adulthood at 18 and 22. I wondered if was absolutely necessary to have a complete hysterectomy.

After visiting with the surgeon, I drove away from the

medical building trembling, tears in my eyes and a longing for comfort or concern from someone, anyone. I longed for the pre-brain injury Perry who would have been with me when the news was delivered, then whispered soothing assurances that I would be okay as he held my hand. I longed for the Perry who would have told me that my essence of womanhood would be intact even if I was missing my uterus and ovaries.

The surgery was carefully timed around availability of help, both for me in the recuperation stage and for caring for Perry at home. With my doctor, we decided on the week after Christmas. Zack would be home for winter break from college. Paul would be on vacation from high school. My aunt Georgina, her husband, and two teenage boys would come while I was in the hospital. My sister Donna and her husband, Philip, were scheduled to come after I was discharged home.

After the surgery, I awoke awash in pain. Hot, searing flashes from the incision below my abdomen made me wince as I stared at the ceiling of my hospital room. I shifted my weight and felt sharp cramps in my pelvic area. I shook myself, trying to rise from the morphine stupor. I drifted in and out of consciousness after the surgery but remembered Georgina's smiling face at the foot of my bed while they wheeled me out of the recovery room.

"You're fine, Cyn! Everything went well! They got it all!"

The mass turned out to be borderline malignant, mostly benign. But why was I in so much pain? Did they not give me enough anesthesia?

"Ow … ouch …help … me … help me."

Was I dreaming or talking in my sleep? I opened my eyes. It wasn't my voice. It was coming from next door. It wasn't a youthful voice but not an elderly one either. It sounded like a woman in her 30s perhaps, maybe 40s, a weak, gravelly voice.

"Help me … Annie! … Ann … nie! Annie … help me!"

Did the woman next door have a hysterectomy, and was she feeling the same pain as me? Why wasn't anyone responding to her?

"Help me, help me, help me!"

A nurse entered the room next door and spoke in soothing tones. "It's okay, it's okay. Try to lift your arm."

"No! No! It hurts! It hurts!" the woman screamed. "MOTHER! MOTHER!"

Mother? Maybe she was younger than I thought. Who was this woman crying for her mother, and what was the matter with her?

I felt a pang of loss, thinking about my mother. I missed the way she stood over me when I was a child, feeling my forehead for signs of fever, concern on her face. I missed having the old Perry next to me, stroking my hand and telling me I was fine. I thought about Perry now, at home. Was he okay? Georgina and her family were there with him, as well as the full-time caregiver. Even in my incapacitated state, there was no escaping my caregiver role, wondering if his needs were met and how he was doing.

I fell asleep again, lost in a morphine fog.

The next time I woke, it was the middle of the night. My pain had subsided and the room was dark. I could hear the moaning sounds of the woman next door through the open door. I wanted to shut the door so I could fall back asleep but was immobilized, still hooked to an IV.

"Help me, help me, help me."

While I wallowed in my own pain, I felt resentful. *Can you give it a rest?* I was in pain too. I wasn't crying out. *How cowardly*, I thought.

In the morning, the nurse was checking on my bandages when her cell phone rang. She lowered her voice, but I heard, "I'm in Room 302, next to the one with the metastases in her breast ... yes, she's a difficult one."

The nurse glanced at me, then stepped outside the room realizing she had compromised the woman's privacy. I felt a stirring of sympathy. A mass in her breast had metastasized. It could have been me, I thought. What if my mass had been cancerous? Would I be moaning like the woman next door? She was experiencing an entirely different kind of pain. Mine was subsiding and would eventually go away. But hers would most likely get worse.

The nursing assistant came in later and got me to stand on my feet. My abdomen and legs were on fire but I was forced to walk to the lavatory and back. After I was left alone, I gave myself more doses of morphine and practiced getting up and tottering around the room. By the second day, I could get up on my own, not needing the help of nursing assistants or morphine.

The woman in the room next door didn't fare as well. In the evening, the nurses tried to turn her over.

"My leg! My leg!" she screamed, her voice echoing up and down the hallway. "Mother! Mother! MOTHER!"

They must have managed to get her in position because her cries subsided. Then there were voices outside my door. *It must be her mother and father and a doctor*, I surmised. The doctor's voice was deep and clear

"The only options right now are surgery or hospice … if hospice, maybe two months. I don't know what you want to do. I don't know if she is strong enough for surgery right now. I don't know if surgery would even help. The cancer has spread."

I felt remorseful for resenting her moaning earlier. She was staring death in the face, with dismal options. I didn't want to hear or know anymore. I remembered the grief and shock of those hours in the intensive care unit, not knowing if Perry would ever awaken or what his state of mind would be if he survived. I didn't want to hear another family's heart rendering decisions. I turned up the TV to drown out the voices in the hallway.

That evening, Perry, Zack and Paul came to visit along with Georgina and Dave and their two sons. For three hours I forgot about the woman next door and her moaning. Perry's face brightened at the sight of me. He stood next to my bed and stroked my hand but I don't think he registered why I was there. We got him to sit on the couch near the window while I ate the fried chicken they brought and the white chocolate cake from my favorite bakery. The chatter of happy voices in the room drowned out the conversations next door.

But later that night I was awakened again.

"Mo…ther! Mo…ther! Mother!"

Another sleepless night ensued. She screamed for Annie again, cried when they tried to move her. I pictured her wrapped in bandages, her legs in traction perhaps. Why was it so difficult and painful to move her leg?

The next day, I expanded my walking to outside of my room. I put on the padded socks and shuffled up and down the hallway, hunched over in my hospital gown. I peered into the room next door as I passed. The curtain was drawn but I caught a glimpse of her parents, a middle-aged couple in their late 50s. After I circled the ward, I got a better view of her parents on my return. The father was trim and athletic with graying hair, dressed in khaki pants and a polo shirt. The mother was plump with rounded cheeks and wearing a red sweatshirt and comfortable walking shoes. They looked solemn as they huddled in conversation with a doctor in a white coat outside the curtain.

My strength was returning. I was able to get up and close my door in the evenings to shut out the constant moaning and the hushed conversations in my doorway. Even though I was facing a recuperation period of six weeks, I looked forward to going home. My health would only get better. Perry would continue to recover also, albeit at a slow, glacial pace. So far, we had evaded the prospect of death.

On discharge day, I sat on the couch next to my bed fully dressed and waited for the nurse to take out the IV, to release me from this world. I tapped my foot in impatience. The nurse was standing outside the door engaged in conversation with the woman's father.

"We don't know what to do … none of the options …" he said, his voice breaking, then dissolving into a sob.

"Whatever you decide to do, we will back you. It's your decision, and they are all tough decisions," said the nurse. "Whatever you decide, we will be here for you."

I wanted to cover my ears to block out the heartbreak. Georgina walked in the door and I was glad to have someone to converse with so I wouldn't have to overhear more of their conversation. At last the nurse brought my discharge papers, a wheelchair was found and I was taken to the car. I winced each time we hit a speed bump which punctuated the pain but I felt a sense of elation of being free from the hospital. *I don't have cancer. I will get better.* As I stared out the windows, I couldn't stop thinking about the woman in the room next door whose face I never glimpsed. Her plaintive cries of pain were etched in my mind. I was going home to heal and recover but for her, the real pain was yet to come.

Chapter 28

━━

In June, three years after Perry's brain injury, I was looking forward to the reunion at Paul's elementary school. Paul had just graduated from high school and his former elementary school organized a reunion before everyone left for college. For many of the children, they had gone from kindergarten through sixth grade together. I had fond memories of conversations with the mothers of Paul's friends when I was a stay-at-home mom and we dropped off or picked up children from each other's houses. Although we did not keep up the connections after our children went to different middle and high schools, I looked forward to catching up with them.

At the reunion, I looked at the young adult faces surrounding me and tried to guess which child that face now belonged to. They looked so mature, so self-confident. We connected with Paul's former teachers and the administrators. Michael's mother approached us and gave me a hug.

"Can you believe we made it through this college application process?" she said. "It was so stressful, getting all the applications done and essays and all."

Paul had handled all of his applications without my help.

He didn't seem overly stressed by it and I was too preoccupied to be of much help.

"It wasn't so bad," I said. "Why was it so stressful? Where is Michael going?"

"Oh, he's going to Harvard but it was just such an ordeal, don't you think?"

I didn't know what to say. To me, an ordeal was sitting in intensive care waiting for your husband to wake from a coma. An ordeal was not knowing how far your husband would come back from brain injury. I was relieved when Danny's mother joined us.

"It's been such a long time since we've seen each other!" she squealed. "How are you? I heard what happened and I think about you all the time."

I hugged her back. "How are you?"

"Oh, I'm so stressed, you know, with graduation and everything. Isn't this stressful?"

"Not really," I said, dumbfounded. "Graduation is a happy thing. What's so stressful?"

She threw up her hands. "You know, this time of year, with all these activities, the after-party, all of that!"

I looked away, my smile frozen on my face. *No,* I wanted to say. *Stressful is worrying about your husband pulling his pants down in a middle of a crowd and worrying that you won't be able to control him or calling health insurance to insist that his therapy get covered.* But graduation from high school? That was not stressful. But what right did I have to ruin my friend's lovely day with my laments?

"Yes, you are so right," I said, as we moved toward a picnic table. "There is so much going on."

After I seated Perry, I went to stand in line at the food table with Danny's mother, who was now engrossed in deep conversation with Sam's father. I caught snippets of what he was saying as I stood behind them.

"…Jonathan Club and this surf machine, then a bucking horse, like in that Debra Winger movie …" He stopped when he saw me and smiled.

"Nice to see you!" he said, shaking my hand. "We were just talking about graduation night and what they did at Sam's school."

Danny's mother turned to me. "What did they do at Paul's school?"

I paused. What did they do? "I think they went to a club in Hollywood. Then bowling and the beach? I don't really know. Paul never gave me the full rundown."

They exchanged knowing glances. I was one of those "out-of-it" mothers, not involved in their kid's activities. But I didn't care. It seemed so frivolous, these children of privilege who partied at the Jonathan Club and would go on to elite colleges and become members of elite clubs themselves. Did it matter if they went to the Jonathan Club or a private club in Hollywood? If Perry hadn't had his heart attack, would I have been just as interested in the details of graduation and the after-party?

In his last two years of high school, Paul often complained about some of the students at his school, how their conversations seemed superficial to him, how their lifestyles were opulent and overdone. I would get annoyed and remind him of how lucky he was to be getting such a good education, remembering my own poor experience at public school.

But that day at the reunion, I finally understood how he felt. We were just trying to survive, trying to put on a brave face and carry on, while around us everyone was worried about things that really didn't matter at all.

CHAPTER 29

—✦—

Two months later in August, Paul left for Bowdoin College in Maine. I had pictured that I would deliver Paul to college, like I had with Zack. But over the summer, Paul and Zack hatched a plan to drive our minivan across the country and share the van on the east coast. They would couch surf along the way, visiting friends. Paul wanted to get in one last backpacking trip in the Sierras before leaving and would fly to Denver after his trip to join Zack for the rest of the drive east.

So instead of accompanying Paul to college, instead of getting him settled and buying him sheets and pillows, instead of crying as I left him in the dorm, all of my sadness and heartache played out at home.

The night before his departure, we lingered over dinner. Paul had cooked his special chicken, coated with bread crumbs and parmesan cheese and lightly sautéed. I tried to savor the meal in spite of the lump in my throat. This was the end of our time together.

"It's been wonderful having you under our roof for these past 18 years," I said, trying to make light of it. "You are such a good son." I didn't trust myself to say more, as I felt myself choking up.

Paul chuckled. "Thanks, Mom."

I turned to Perry. "Paul is leaving for college tomorrow. What do you think? Do you want to say something to him?"

Perry stopped chewing and put down his fork. He looked at Paul, his eyes wide. "Good job, Paul!" he said in a clear, deep voice.

In the morning, as we got ready to leave for the airport, Paul climbed onto our bed and crouched next to Perry.

"Goodbye, Dad, I'm going off to college," he whispered.

Perry was in deep sleep. He stirred, then pulled the blanket over his head.

I fought back tears, remembering all the mornings when Paul was a toddler and would climb into our bed after waking early, then snuggle between the two us. He would fall asleep again, his tiny body nestled between ours. Even as he grew older, he loved to jump onto our bed on weekend mornings and ask, "What are we doing today?" That chapter was over.

At the airport, I sobbed as I hugged him goodbye. He gathered his duffel bag and backpack and started to walk away. Then he stopped, turned back and hugged me again.

"You'll be fine, Mom. Remember when I went to HMI?"

I nodded, not trusting my voice to speak.

I cried during the entire drive to my office downtown, knowing that this was not at all like when he went to HMI. Then, I knew he was coming back, he would be living at home again for his senior year, he was not yet an adult. Now, his leaving meant that my mothering days were over. It wouldn't ever be the same, the feeling of protecting, nurturing and worrying about him, knowing where he went and when he would come home. The days of planned meals together, making sure he had his homework done or enough money in his wallet were over. He and Zack would come back for visits and maybe stay for a few weeks or months or between jobs but it would not be the same. I had cupped them in the palm of my hands all these years then gently let go, watching them fly away. My heart broke a little each time they left.

IF PERRY MISSED PAUL, HE never expressed it to me. To him, life went on as usual. The boys were there and not there. When they were home, he always looked at them with wonder and pride, happy to see them. When they were gone, he didn't ask about them.

"What do you miss the most about Perry?" Nancy, my neighbor once asked me.

Without hesitation, I said, "I miss the conversation. Perry used to call me several times a day. He always asked about my day, what I was doing."

I remembered that much of our relationship was grounded in talk and conversation, about our day, of mundane things of who said what, funny anecdotes, things that troubled us, pesky personnel, testy encounters with others. We talked when we felt buoyant or insecure, anxious or worried about a current project. We talked about our favorite topic, our children, and what we hoped for them in the future, things they had said or done in the last day, what their schedules were. I missed that conversation with my best friend, the person who knew me best and always propped me up, who believed in my abilities with unconditional praise and love.

As I was telling all of this to Nancy, I realized then that Paul had become my conversationalist in the last few years. After he had come back from HMI, he was more inquisitive and talkative. During dinner, I would tell him about what happened that day, how difficult it was to manage people, what aggravations I faced working in a large bureaucracy. As time went on, it became a nightly ritual to hear about Paul's day, stories from school or his courses, or what bothered him. Then I would tell him about the characters at work, the latest political struggles and eventually, he began asking about my day, wanting to hear the latest.

My chest tightened. In a subtle and gradual way, he had

become my confidant, and now he was gone.

OUR EVENINGS WERE MUCH QUIETER after Paul left for college. There wasn't much conversing with Perry at dinner. He didn't remember what he had done that day so I didn't ply him with questions. He didn't ask about my day or what I did at work. My job no longer consisted of detailed analysis work where I could hole up in my cubicle and work numbers. My days were now filled with meetings and constant interaction, either face to face or on the phone. Now when I came home, I found comfort in the silence that greeted me. So it was pleasant, peaceful even, to have a silent dinner. I read the paper or a magazine while I waited for him to finish.

One evening, I made finger foods for dinner—roasted cauliflower, tator tots, baked chicken pieces. When Perry liked my cooking, he ate with no distraction. He had just finished the chicken on his plate.

"Would you like more chicken?" I asked.

"Later," he whispered.

"Why are you whispering?"

"Because it's so quiet in here."

"Do you like it quiet?" I asked.

He leaned back and closed his eyes and didn't answer, but I knew what his answer was. I liked the quietness, too. I found it comforting.

Chapter 30

～✺～

Years before his brain injury, Perry had promised to take me to Tofino on the western edge of Vancouver Island in British Columbia for storm watching on my 50th birthday.

"I love the rain, I love storms, wouldn't this be fun?" I said, showing Perry an article on the Wickaninnish Inn.

He scanned the magazine and looked at the pictures. "Yes, that looks really nice. We'll go for your 50th and make it special."

But as my 50th birthday approached, I knew Perry was never going to "take" me anywhere again. It had seemed like a lifetime ago, that promise. I remembered whispering in his ear when he was in a coma, "Come back to me, wake up, we have so many more things to do. We have to take our baby Paul to Rome, you have to take me to Tofino."

He woke up, but the Perry that came back was not the same.

"We'll take you to Tofino," said Zack.

"Let's all go," said Paul. "It's your 50th birthday, we should have a big celebration."

My research showed that getting to Tofino was not an easy

task. Although we had traveled to the East Coast with Perry numerous times by now and had taken long road trips with him, we had not embarked on a trip quite this challenging. It required a flight to Vancouver, then a ferry to Vancouver Island and another four-hour drive to the west coast of the island.

"No problem," said Zack. "You'll have me and Paul to help. No sweat."

After days of studying flight schedules, time tables for ferries, car rental rates and researching hotels, I was overwhelmed by all the details. It seemed so complicated but I broke our travel into manageable segments: Vancouver, ferry to Victoria, drive to Tofino, then ferry back to Vancouver before catching a flight home.

WITH ZACK AND PAUL ON hand, traveling with Perry was much easier. They helped in the security lines, baggage and boarding. During our stay in Vancouver, we walked to the beach, shopped along the stores on Robson, visited the anthropology museum and explored Stanley Park with plenty of rest periods back at the hotel. The ferry to Victoria was smooth and comfortable. While waiting for the ferry at the Tsawassen terminal, we browsed the booths selling clothing, toys, watches, sunglasses and gourmet fudge. We chose from an assortment of restaurants selling crepes, sausages, sandwiches and coffee. Best of all, there was a large, clean family restroom where I could take care of Perry.

We kept an eye on the weather for our drive to Tofino. I hadn't calculated that in order to drive somewhere for storm-watching, I would have to drive through inclement weather. The boys were not yet 25 and I didn't feel comfortable letting them drive the rental car, which meant I was the sole driver.

I was terrified of driving in snow and ice after I once spun out on black ice outside of Flagstaff, Arizona while we were in college. Whenever there was a hint of snow or ice or even excessive rain, I surrendered the wheel to Perry. But now, there was no one to surrender the driving to.

I clutched the steering wheel in a tight grip as we left Victoria under threatening skies that turned into torrential rains by the time we reached Nanaimo. The sun came out briefly when we stopped for lunch. We entered dense forest as we headed toward Port Alberni. Strong winds blew branches off of trees, littering the road. I tightened my grip on the wheel as we climbed over a low pass near the Mackenzie range and a light snow began to fall. I prayed that we would not slide or have to put on chains. Once over the pass, the snow turned to rain, then hail as I inched along, tense and nervous. By the time we dropped to sea level after Kennedy Lake, we hit high winds, hail and then snow as we pulled into the driveway of the Wickaninnish Inn.

We had arrived during a gale force storm. After we checked into our rooms, I let out a big sigh of relief. We had made it. Our room had big sliding glass doors overlooking the Pacific and furious waves pounded the rocks outside our window. The wind whistled as sleet and snow seemed to fall sideways. I kicked off my shoes and grabbed Perry's hands, facing him. I jumped up and down in a happy jig.

"Wow, look at this," I shouted. "This is exactly what I wanted!"

He laughed at my delight and tried to jump with me then swung my hands side to side. We lit a fire and I spent the rest of the afternoon gazing at the thrashing waves whipped by the wind and the snow collecting on the railing of the balcony until it became too dark to see.

THE STORM LEFT TWO FEET of snow the next morning. As we set off to explore the island, I was nervous about driving in the snow. Although the highway had been plowed, many of the side roads leading to trails were still closed. I took a wrong turn onto a narrow road, down a hill leading to the water. Halfway down the hill, I realized we had driven into the village settlement of the local Native Americans. This was not the state park. I made a U turn to go back up the hill but the back wheels spun on the icy road. We were stuck.

I turned to the boys in the back seat. "What do we do now?" None of us had experience with driving in the snow. I turned to Perry. "What should we do?"

He had his eyes closed and shook his head from side to side. "I don't know," he said.

I revved the engine again and the wheels continued to spin. Then we heard a yell from a window of the house up the driveway to our left.

"Use your floormats!"

Puzzled, Paul stepped out of the car.

"Hey buddy, use your floormats on the back tires!" said an older man with dark black hair from his open window upstairs.

Paul reached into the car and took out the floor mat from the back seat and placed it under the back tire. I revved the engine again and we picked up enough traction to get forward momentum up the hill. Paul raced back for the floor mat and gave our helpers a thank you wave.

WE DIDN'T ENCOUNTER ANY MORE big storms during our stay at the Wickaninnish Inn, which provided some relief for me. I was worried about driving back to Nanaimo and encountering icy roads. I checked weather updates and asked the front desk for the latest road conditions constantly. We took an easy hike in the state park, lunched in the tiny hamlet at Ucelet, huddled in our rooms over pizza and enjoyed the view. It wasn't as adventurous or active as we would have traveled pre-brain injury but I was content.

The drive back to Nanaimo was smooth, there was no ice, no snow as we passed deep, glacial lakes, craggy peaks and redwood forests. On our last night in Vancouver, we had a celebratory dinner on Granville Island, overlooking the Vancouver skyline. I felt a sense of accomplishment, a new-found strength. We had made it to Tofino for my 50th birthday.

CHAPTER 31

⁓⫫⁓

Later that summer, on a sunny June day, Perry and I went to the Century City mall at five in the afternoon. He hated shopping, but always sat patiently and obediently while I tried on clothes. That afternoon, he resisted as we started to enter Ann Taylor.

"I just want to browse," I said.

"No, I want to stay outside," he said.

I hesitated. I usually brought him into the stores with me, then sat him in a chair while I shopped. A month before, we had gone to New York for Zack's graduation and he sat on a couch for over an hour in Bloomingdales. I checked on him every 20 minutes. But on this day, I gave in and sat him on bench outside.

"I will just be ten minutes, okay?" I said. He nodded yes.

Ten minutes later, I returned to the bench. Perry was gone. Where was he? I looked around. He didn't walk very fast. I circled the area near the bench, looking for his shuffle step, his hunched form. My pulse quickened. He had never gotten up by himself before, no matter where I seated him. I widened my search to the walking areas around the mall, making loops until I covered all the outdoor areas. My heart raced. Where could he have gone? I walked in loops around the mall again, panic rising in me. Maybe he moved to another bench. I searched all the benches outside.

Thirty minutes had gone by and there was no sign of him. I found a security guard and tried to quell the panic in my voice as I blurted, "I can't find my husband, he's brain injured, he has no short term memory and he has trouble balancing. He wandered away."

"What does he look like?" the guard asked, raising his radio to ask for help.

Oh God. What did I put on him this morning? "He's wearing khaki shorts. A dark green polo shirt. Brown hair, balding, brown eyes, five feet seven." *What else? Which cap did I put on his head?* "He's wearing a baseball cap, grey or dark green. I can't remember. White socks. White tennis shoes," I said, my voice shaking.

"Okay, I'll get my partner and we'll search this side of the mall," he said. "You search the other side or stay near the bench in case he comes back."

I walked quickly, almost running, as I looked in every store on my way back to the bench. Nothing. *Where is he? Could he have followed someone?*

Another thirty minutes passed. I saw the security guard and rushed toward him.

"We didn't find him," he said. "I've called Los Angeles Police and they are sending someone."

In minutes, I was reciting the same story to a uniformed officer who was taking notes. "Do you have a picture of him?" he asked.

"No," I said as my mind went through the contents of my purse. I didn't even have his wallet with me. He didn't have a medic bracelet because he never wore jewelry. He didn't even wear a wedding ring. Before his brain injury, he took off his watch the moment he came home from work. In the hospital, he would tear off the ID tags from his wrists whenever he could.

"We'll check around the perimeter of the mall, then drive to your house to see if maybe someone gave him a ride home. Does he have a house key?"

"No," I said. He didn't have anything on him, no identification, no house key, nothing.

I didn't know what to do next. *The car. Maybe he went down to the car.* I took the escalator down to the garage in case he may have gone downstairs, my heart pounding. But with his faulty memory, there was no way he would remember where we parked or even which car belonged to us. He wasn't at the car. I searched the aisles next to where we parked. No Perry. How could he have just disappeared into thin air? It was now after 6;00, dinnertime. He was probably hungry. His diaper was probably wet.

What if he's trying to walk home? I could search the streets near the mall, drive the route home to see if I could spot him. The security guards were still searching upstairs. I got in the car and as I drove down Olympic, my cell phone rang. My heart jumped. Maybe they found him, maybe it was the security guard at the mall or the police. But it was Zack, calling from New York. He was getting ready to move to New Mexico for an art internship. He needed me to look up something at home.

"I can't, Zack! I've lost your dad!" I cried into the phone. I pulled over onto a side street and sobbed as I told him about the searches underway, how I was driving around the neighborhood.

"Who is there with you?" he asked.

"No one, it's just me and your dad. Paul is backpacking in the Sierras," I said.

"You shouldn't be alone. Who is in L.A. that can help you?" he asked.

"Manny and Nancy are in Santa Barbara. I don't know who to call."

"Go back to the mall," he said. "He's got to be there. He's never wandered away before. I'm going to make some calls to find people to help you."

Before I could respond, Zack hung up. I was engulfed in helplessness. *What do I do now?* I went back to the mall and found the security guard again. There was still no sign of Perry, although they were still searching. I paced the mall in circles again and again. In the next hour, friends appeared: Orly and Ed, from our college days, then Rich, from the law firm, then Manny, Nancy and David, who were on their way home from Santa Barbara when Zack called them. For the next few hours, I didn't feel so alone but my panic did not subside. We searched every corner of the mall, the men going into every restroom stall, the security guards searching the movie theaters as darkness fell. We searched the hotel nearby, looked at the deserted plaza in front of the dark and empty office towers. There was so sign of Perry. Where could he be in the dark?

Near midnight, I don't remember what else was said or how it was decided that the search was over. We had looked in every corner, every square inch of the mall. He was not there. The police had been to the house but found it empty and dark. I was escorted home in my car by Nancy, my mind consumed by nightmares. *Where is Perry? He's wandering this city still, in the dark.* He must be confused, agitated. He must be wondering where I was. What if someone had abducted him? I was beside myself with worry.

At home, Rich suggested we contact the media to alert the public. I needed to call the police again to check on their status. Someone else suggested calling the emergency rooms of hospitals and I got on the phone immediately, to Cedars, St. Johns, Santa Monica. He was not at any of them. Where could he be? I was about to call the police again when I scrolled through the phone log to see if there were any missed calls. There were two from an unfamiliar 310 area code and the label read, "Century City Ho." My heart lurched. Did they find him at the Century City Hotel? I called the number and got connected to the Century City Hospital, a small facility tucked in a corner of the office complex. I described Perry and explained about the missed call, my voice shaking.

"Yes, we have him here," said the man on the phone. "Paramedics brought him in earlier this evening, about eight. He was disoriented and had no ID but he gave us his name and his home phone number. We called but no one answered and we didn't leave a message."

Relief like I had never known flooded through me. While we were searching in the dark, he was at the hospital, being cared for. Nancy and I jumped in the car and raced to the hospital where we found Perry in bed, in a gown, hooked to IV's.

"Perry, I was so worried about you!" I said as I rushed to his side. "Are you okay?"

He turned to look at me and flashed his brilliant smile. "I'm fine," he said.

"Did you know you were lost?" I asked.

"No, I'm not lost," he said. He seemed calm and rested.

"They found him on the corner of Balsalm and Holmby," said the nurse. That intersection was a few blocks from the mall, but on the streets that curved and turned. No wonder I couldn't find him when I was searching the streets. "He was lying on someone's lawn and they called the paramedics. He was dehydrated but he's in good condition now."

"Are you ready to go home?" I asked.

He looked at me with eyes filled with love and smiled. If he had been traumatized by the experience, it was not apparent from his demeanor. I felt stabbed by regret. Why didn't I just insist that he come into Ann Taylor with me? What was I thinking, leaving him on a bench outside the store? I wanted to throw myself at his feet and say, *I'm sorry. I'm sorry I didn't take care of you, I'm sorry I failed you in this most basic way.* He looked at me with complete trust to lead him and take care of him and I was filled with remorse. I thought of all the times I left him for a few minutes, out of my view—at the airport while I went to the bathroom, in Bloomingdales in New York—what if this had happened then? I thought of all the challenges we had faced so far, his bouts of agitation, his incontinence, his silence and unresponsiveness. All of those challenges had been solvable in the end or I had found a way to make it work, to keep it under control. But nothing had prepared me for losing Perry, and I knew I couldn't do it again.

Since that day, Perry has never been out of sight of me or the caregiver. We put a wallet in his pocket with a photocopy of his ID and emergency numbers. We considered a medic alert bracelet, but he would not wear it. He has never wandered away again but that day was a reminder that I could never let my guard down, that I had to be vigilant and on alert at all times. I have never forgotten that feeling on that June day, the despair, the helplessness, the feeling that I was a complete failure as a caregiver, the feeling of being without Perry. I had almost lost him once, due to circumstances beyond my control. I would not lose him based on something I *could* control.

CHAPTER 32

-ᴗᴥᴗ-

In August of 2007, the boys wanted to throw us a 25th anniversary party. I resisted. It felt like a travesty after all we had been through with his brain injury. This was not how I envisioned our 25th year of marriage would be like. Was Perry even cognizant of the significance or would it be an exercise in sorrow and pity, reminding us of what was lost?

I thought back to our wedding day. Nothing about our wedding followed tradition because we wanted to break free of the rituals my sisters and brother dutifully followed in their weddings—the bridal showers, registering for gifts and china place settings, the escorting of the bride down the aisle, the special knife to cut the wedding cake, the little wedding favors. We found the Brazilian Room, a rustic lodge set amidst the meadows and hills dotted with oak trees in Tilden Park in Berkeley. There was no line of bridesmaids and ushers, just us, a best man and maid of honor. I didn't need my brother to escort me down the aisle; I was an independent woman and walked on my own, unaccompanied. Our vows were devoid of any language about "obeying," and the actual ceremony was so brief that when my grandfather arrived fifteen minutes late, it was over and the guests had already erupted in applause after our kiss.

We had hired an amateur photographer who had never done a wedding so we got hundreds of pictures of the trio playing classical music on the flagstone patio and very few shots of the reception inside, the wedding party or our families after the ceremony. The photographer also discovered, too late, that his flash didn't work.

Following Chinese tradition, the women in my family gave me jade and gold jewelry for the wedding. My mother wanted me to wear all the jewelry I had received at the reception after the ceremony. I resisted, not wanting to follow any traditions but on the day of the wedding, I gave in and let her adorn me with jewelry. Perry's favorite picture was of me standing on the patio after the ceremony, with flowers in my short hair, my ivory Victorian style gown with lace sleeves and collar, a modest smile on my face, wearing a gold bracelet on each wrist and three jade necklaces over the lace of the gown.

I looked over those pictures now and thought back to how reluctant we had been to make a big deal of our wedding. We got married when he finished law school had accepted the job with the law firm. The words "boyfriend" and "girlfriend" didn't adequately describe what we meant to each other. There was no proposal, no engagement ring. We just knew that we wanted to spend the rest of our lives together.

My sisters got excited and fawned over the details of the wedding. They wrapped Jordan almonds in dark blue netting with printed ribbons that said, "Perry and Cynthia, August 15, 1982" because I was going to have irises as my wedding flower. When I found out irises were not in bloom in August and I would have to pick Peruvian lilies, they undid all the wrapped almonds, retied them in pink netting and reprinted pink ribbons. My sister Rosemary made sure we had a special knife to cut the cake, found me a garter to wear and for Perry to toss. It wasn't until years later that I realized weddings weren't just about the two of us. It was for all our family and friends.

So I gave in to the boys and let them plan the anniversary party. Paul designed an invitation with a picture of us from our wedding, glasses of champagne held up for a toast. My sisters wanted to know about the décor for the party. RSVP's began trickling in. Zack was coming back from his art internship in New Mexico, my brother was coming from Livermore, my sisters from Salinas. Paul scanned old photos to put into a slide show. On the day of the party, my siblings came early to help set up the rented tables and chairs in the backyard and string Japanese lanterns across the patio. Pink Peruvian lilies decorated the tables, just like they did 25 years ago.

It was a warm, balmy Saturday evening when our 50 or so guests gathered in the backyard. For once, the Westside was not shrouded in fog. After mojitos and beer, we dined on pasta and salad from our favorite Italian restaurant. Perry seemed alert and responsive as guests chatted with him.

After dinner, Paul stretched a white sheet across the garage door and played his slide show. I smiled at the sight of us in college, with my waist length hair and gauze shirt, Perry with his shoulder-length wispy hair and Earth shoes. For the next seven minutes, the pictures ran through a progression of our years together, us holding trout in the Sierras, us arm-in-arm as Perry graduated law school, our wedding, then both of us with short hair holding Zack as a baby, then Paul. Another set of pictures showed the four of us together, always in the outdoors, the same beaming smile from Perry. The frames of the pictures flowed seamlessly and I didn't even notice when the photos transitioned to Perry after his brain injury. What stayed with me was his smile and his eyes, lively and full of love as he gazed at me.

IN THE WEEKS PRIOR TO the party, Geri, his speech therapist, had worked with Perry to prepare a speech. After the lights were turned on again, Perry stood in front of the garage door facing our guests and in a soft voice, read from the piece of paper he had dictated to Geri. We gathered close to hear.

the corner. As he spotted me, his face broke out in a wide grin. I reached to hug him. We had made it! We were in Istanbul together!

As our cab squeezed through the narrow entrance to the Sultanahmet, I was filled with wonder. Near the Blue Mosque with its six minarets, the cab let us out at the hotel. The call to prayer blared from loudspeakers, filling the air with its mournful sound. After dropping our bags, we walked around the exterior of the Blue Mosque, then the Haghia Sophia, to get our bearings.

The next morning Zack woke with a fever. My heart sank in disappointment. These days of freedom from caregiving were so precious, so hard to find. Should I sit in the hotel and watch him sleep? I got him breakfast and found a pharmacy with aspirin, then set out to explore the Sultanahmet on my own.

I felt self-conscious walking alone, not sure of where I was going. I found the elliptical track of the Hippodrome and studied the three obelisks in the center, one from the 10th century. I stepped into the courtyard of the Blue Mosque and admired the carvings on the stone, the massive wooden doors but wanted to wait to visit the inside until Zack felt better.

I strolled to the Basilica Cisterns, the Yerebatan Sarnici, built in A.D. 537 by Emperor Justinian during the Byzantine Empire. After descending the stairs, I stood gazing at the Roman columns in the semi-darkness, with Turkish music playing in the background. The chilly January air was even colder underground and I shivered in my down jacket. I followed the dark paths through the cistern, to the far northeast end to see the Medusa heads. There were few visitors and I felt scared wandering alone. When I reached the first Medusa head with hair carved like snakes, I shuddered. Would I turn to stone if I gazed too long? Who would notice?

I was thankful when a group of Japanese tourists arrived. I hovered near them for comfort while I walked to the next Medusa head. As I headed toward the exit, I felt a deep sense of loneliness. If Perry, the old Perry, was there, he would hold my hand. Even the new Perry would have gripped my hand tightly and I wouldn't have felt so alone.

I checked back at the hotel to see how Zack was faring. He was still feverish and sleepy. There was no way he was getting up to go sightseeing.

I decided to take a Turkish bath. I entered the Cagaloglu Hamam, built in 1741, the last one built during the Ottoman Empire. I was given a cubicle to undress in, then tied a pestemal, a Turkish wrap, around my body and stepped into slippery wooden sandals. A woman guided me to the steam room, threw a couple of bowls of warm water over me and gestured for me to lie down on the marble in the middle of the room. The sun shining through the Roman arches and dome gave it a feeling of light. I lay on my stomach on the marble slab for five, then ten minutes, then turned over onto my back. I was the only person in the bathing room.

My mind wandered. What was I doing here? What was my place in this world? I wondered how Perry was doing. Did he miss me? After twenty minutes, I got anxious. Where was that woman? I realized how vulnerable I was, completely naked on a marble slab in a foreign country and not knowing the language.

Another ten minutes went by before the woman came back, wearing a black swimsuit. She filled a pail with hot water then walked toward me, gesturing for me to get up. I stood and she threw water over the slab of marble, then motioned for me to lay down on my back. With a loofah cloth, she scrubbed my body, pulling my arm to my chest so that I could feel the dead skin that had been rubbed off. She gestured for me to turn over and scrubbed my back. Then she rinsed my body with bowls of steaming hot water and began the soap massage, pounding on my lower and upper back then the back of my knees. Finally, she led me to the basin, told me to sit between her legs while she shampooed my hair. I felt like a baby being handled and scrubbed while she massaged the top of my head, then my face. My eyes were closed as she poured hot water all over to rinse. I opened my eyes and felt purged of my nervousness and insecurity.

I walked back to the hotel, glowing and completely relaxed. I didn't even feel bothered by the Turkish rug dealers who tried to entice me every ten feet. Zack was still ailing and it didn't seem like a good idea to get him outside in the cold January weather. After an hour rest, I decided to visit the Haghia Sophia, a short distance from our hotel. I was breathless as I entered the dome; the scale was more stupendous than what I had read. I walked up the winding, worn cobblestone path to the upper gallery and felt a sense of loss and loneliness again. Couples held hands, families walked together, tour groups bunched around their guide. I walked alone, untethered but clinging to memories of what once was, of a family and a husband intact.

I rubbed the worn surface of the railing in the upper gallery. It had probably been touched by Roman Emperors and Ottoman Sultans hundreds of years before me. Instead of feeling divine, I was filled with doubt. What was I doing here all alone?

The next day, Mary Beth, the mother of one of Zack's former roommates came to visit. She was teaching English at a university forty-five minutes away and stayed with us for two days. Under Mary Beth's guidance, we were swept into a whirlwind of activity as she taught us how to navigate the city. We took a boat up the Golden Horn to visit the mosque at Eyup, we boarded the tram that took us from the Sultanahmet to Beyoglu on the European side. We walked across the Galata Bridge and ate fish sandwiches straight from fisherman's nets. We shopped in the Spice Bazaar, examined the fierce models of soldiers and watched the Mehter Band perform at the Military Museum. We drank tea at sunset along the Bosphorus outside the Dolmabache Palace, then strolled Istiklal Caddesi along with crowds on their evening promenade. I found a kindred soul in Mary Beth and caught a glimpse of what travel could be like with someone other than the old Perry.

After she left, Zack and I filled the rest of our days with more sightseeing, a ferry to the Asian side to admire the food market, a tour of the Topkapi Palace, a rainy afternoon at the Anthropology museum and shopping in the Grand Bazaar. By the end of seven days, I had grown accustomed to the muezzin's call for prayer and savored my hot Turkish tea, served in curved glasses. I wasn't filled with longing or loneliness or missing Perry. This was what travel was like on my own, and it felt glorious.

WHEN I RETURNED HOME, PERRY was glad to see me. His face lit up when he saw me and he pursed his lips for a kiss. But he had no conception of how much time had passed.

"Did you know I was gone for ten days?" I asked him.

"Yes," he said, his eyes opened wide.

"Did you miss me? Did you know where I was?" I asked.

"I thought you died," he said. Then he broke into a laugh.

"He did not," said Paul. "I didn't tell him where you were because I didn't want to get him confused. He was fine. He didn't think you were dead."

I was unnerved in any case. Did it even make a difference whether I was there in his life or not? For him, life went on as usual. He had no conception of what I did in Istanbul, there was no conversing, no sharing of stories. The first two nights I was home, he held onto me tightly in bed, not wanting to let go.

"Okay, let go of me now, let me sleep," I said. He would release his grip but after five minutes, he would roll towards me again, wrapping his arm across my chest. He burrowed his head into my shoulder, creating a sore spot as my neck stiffened. *How like my life*, I thought, trapped in this uncomfortable position, wanting to escape or move but immobilized, drawn to his warmth.

CHAPTER 34

～╲╱～

Five years after Perry's brain injury, work became more stressful. I received another promotion and now supervised an entire division of more than 100 staff and was given more responsibility. The school district was faced with massive deficits and we had to cut staff. My days were spent in meetings agonizing over how to save jobs and I rarely had a moment alone to concentrate or collect my thoughts. My home was my only refuge and I looked forward to our silent dinners and Perry's ever-present smile. I wanted my home to be a sanctuary; a soothing and consoling environment after a stressful day of work. I wanted it to be a comfortable place for caregiving, a house that would accommodate us into old age.

But the house did not feel restful when I got home. I had too many books crammed into mismatched bookcases. Our small master bedroom retained heat from the afternoon sun and the miniscule closet where I crammed my clothes and shoes was overflowing. The house was not conducive for caregiving and disability, either. The plastic shower bench barely fit in the bathtub in our single full bathroom. The linoleum near the tub warped because water leaked from the shower curtain as we assisted Perry with bathing. The narrow space near the sink meant we had to squeeze around Perry when we helped him shave. The front steps to the house were at a sharp incline and hard for him to keep his balance.

When we had moved in twenty years ago, we knew the house was too small. But we were lulled by the stately camphor trees that lined the L- shaped street, the tidy green lawns and the quietness of the neighborhood. I liked the enclosed backyard where the boys could set up a Slip and Slide. After a few years, we enlarged the tiny den that served as Paul's room when he was an infant, then became my study when I wrote my dissertation. Then we gutted and remodeled the kitchen, brightening it with maple cabinets and white appliances. When the boys hit their teens, we tore down the garage and built a new structure with an all-purpose room on the second story.

Before Perry's brain injury, we had considered remodeling the house again to create more space, but he was reluctant to make another large investment in the house. "Why not move to a bigger house?" he would always say. But we didn't want to leave the camaraderie among our neighbors or the annual Fourth of July block party and winter holiday tea party. We had planted roots in our Mar Vista neighborhood.

I decided to work with an architect to see how we could add more space and build accommodations for disability. For months, I combed over plans with her, arranging rooms like puzzle pieces. At last, we viewed the final blueprints, satisfied. We would expand the three quarter bathroom in the back to include a walk-in shower, the den would be pushed out to add larger closet and become our master bedroom. All the ceilings would be raised and the existing bathroom rearranged to include a separate shower and bathtub. I liked the idea of keeping the one story structure intact, foreseeing a time in the future when stairs would prove to be an obstacle in old age. Construction would take at least eight months due to the extensive work and we would need to move out entirely.

MONTHS BEFORE CONSTRUCTION STARTED, I began culling through our belongings. What could be stored in the room above the garage? What could I get rid of? As I emptied the contents of drawers and closets, I dredged up memories from a past life, vacation photos, postcards and letters from family and old friends, souvenirs from Catalina Island and Washington D.C. They filled me with longing for what our lives used to be. Under the bed, I found dusty shoe boxes with dress shoes for law firm functions and several long cylinders with Perry's fly fishing poles. It was as if they were from another life.

I surveyed the contents of our already crowded garage. It was a repository of our former lives, of dreams no longer possible. There was the box with Perry's waders that he used to wear fly fishing in the high Sierra lakes. Three large canvas bags, lined with plastic slots and drawers to hold his fishing equipment, sat on a shelf, the zippers rusted and covered in a white powder like mold. His mountain bike, bought a month before his heart attack, was propped in the back. A full-sized red canoe, overturned, rested on the top shelf in the back of garage, the foam seats and paddles stuffed underneath. These relics had lain dormant for six years now.

I sifted through boxes of camping equipment, sleeping bags and foam pads. We were not likely to ever go camping again. I found the orange Gregory day pack that Perry bought while we were in college. He carried it on a snow camping trip to Pear Lake with his college buddies and later used it for fishing equipment and old sneakers for wading. I opened the pack, which smelled of mold. His dirt-covered sneakers were still there. With a heavy heart, I threw out old foam pads, water containers, and plastic ponchos, sticky with age. It was time to shed these constant reminders of what used to be and time to start anew.

I NEEDED TO FIND A place to live for the next eight months. "Treat this like a vacation and live in a different part of the city," suggested Georgina. A whole new world opened up with that thought. I looked at apartments near the water, in the marina. Perry and I could go on long walks along the channels, we could gaze at boats from our windows, we wouldn't have to worry about lawns and gardeners and taking out our garbage cans every week. We found a spacious, modern apartment with two bedrooms, two full bathrooms and a huge living room with a wall of windows overlooking boats in the marina. We could smell the sea air from the balcony on the third floor.

As moving day drew near, our house emptied as I moved all my books to the room above the garage. I hired a professional organizer to help with packing and supervising the move. The last night in the house, all our possessions were sealed into packing boxes as our footsteps echoed in the empty rooms. I had a moment of panic. Was I doing the right thing? It was too late to back out now, everything was in motion. Perry had always been the one who handled all home improvement jobs. In our previous remodeling projects, he answered the contractor's questions about joists, permits, and drops for electricity and gas lines. But this time it would be my decision alone on whether we had brushed nickel or polished chrome door hinges, glass or ceramic tiles. Was I going to be able to handle all this?

I reached for the scissors in the kitchen and remembered that everything was already packed. All of our drinking cups were packed too so I couldn't get a glass of ice water. Then I worried about how disorienting this would be for Perry, to move to an entirely new place without any memory of why we were moving in the first place. Was it wise to gut the house of everything that was familiar to someone with no short-term memory? Would I be wiping away even more memories?

IN THE APARTMENT, THERE WAS more space than we'd had for the past twenty years. It took several days to unpack and set up the apartment but after everything was put away, I was disoriented. My possessions were there but it didn't feel like home. I missed my wall of bookshelves, my Shalako from the Zuni reservation, my Steuben glass bowl with the glass candies. What defined the feeling of home, the sense of comfort that comes from home? I wanted to reach for Dominique Browning's *Around the House and In the Garden*, which used to be on the shelf in the kitchen. I wanted to browse through my book of essays about home that described the essence that I missed so much. But everything was packed away, stacked in boxes in the room above the garage.

The following weekend, we went by the house to inspect the progress. A huge dumpster filled the driveway. The ceiling had been taken out in the living room, the entry way closet was gone. The walls separating the main bathroom and the den were demolished. I looked at the bare, gutted walls of the bathroom from the den. Without the ceiling, I could see up to the rafters, to the opening at the side of the roof where the vent opened. I felt a wave of anxiety envelop me. It felt like home but wasn't our home anymore. Without furniture and in its demolished state, the house looked ragged and forlorn. How did this feel to Perry? He was silent with a blank expression on his face as he picked at a loose piece of tarpaper. What if I had made a terrible mistake?

On one of our first weekends in the marina, we walked to the Mermaid Café, a mere 150 yards from our apartment building. Perry hesitated as we left the stairwell and stepped outside. I took his hand and guided him toward the water where there was a railing he could grip. In the past few months, he had lost his balance more often and sometimes just stopped walking. We tried a cane for several weeks, but Perry wasn't able to use it to leverage his balance. On this morning, he gripped my hands, squeezed them tightly, then pulled my arm down, making me off balance.

"Stop it, Perry, just walk forward," I said.

He took two steps, then stopped, gripped my hands and pulled. I tried to steer him towards the handrail near the water but he resisted.

"What is it Perry, why won't you walk?"

He looked at me, eyes wide, not speaking, as if he was in a daze. I pulled him forward and he shuffle stepped, leaning forward at an angle. If I quickened our pace, he lost his balance. He squeezed my fingers so tight that my rings dug into my flesh, making me cry out and drop his hand. He swayed, as if he was going to fall. It took us fifteen minutes to walk those 150 yards. In moving to the marina, I had visions of us taking long walks along the fingers of the marina, exploring all the pathways that led to the main channel. How was I to know that he would have this much difficulty walking? It was as if he was afraid of the water.

"Maybe I should get a wheelchair," I said to Nancy the next day. "I could push Perry around the marina, the walkways are flat and it should be easy enough."

"Great idea," she said. "We used a wheelchair when we traveled with my dad and it was so much easier. We didn't have to worry about his walking or getting winded."

I could use the wheelchair when we traveled in airports or at the mall or when I wanted to cover a lot of ground but got tired of him pulling on my arm. I wanted the feeling of walking at a normal pace again, of being able to go long distances unhindered. But part of me felt that getting a wheelchair meant defeat, that I was no longer invested in rehabilitation and recovery.

I asked Perry, "What do you think of using a wheelchair?"

"No," he said, frowning. "I don't need a wheelchair."

Arnold, his caregiver, was alarmed also. "But he's walking. Why use a wheelchair?"

I had to admit it was for selfish reasons. It was really for me, I wanted my freedom. I ordered a lightweight, foldable wheelchair and weeks later, I pushed Perry past Mother's Beach, then curved around Palawan Way. The March breeze was cool but not too cold. I inhaled the misty ocean air and took long strides, kicked out my legs with each step and stretched my muscles as I moved at a fast clip. It was exhilarating to be walking briskly again, moving at a normal pace even though I was pushing 165 pounds in a wheelchair. The muscles in my arms strained and my palms and fingers tingled from gripping the handlebars but I felt an overwhelming sense of lightness and freedom. There was no more waiting for Perry to catch up with his shuffle step, no worrying about his balance or how far he could walk. I leaned forward to see Perry's expression.

"What do you think, Perry? Is it fun riding in this wheelchair with me pushing you?"

"Whee!" he said as he smiled and tilted his face upward to feel the wind.

CHAPTER 35

⁓⁂⁓

In November, nine months after we moved to the marina, our remodeled home was ready. One Saturday morning after we moved back, I wandered the house, feeling content as I admired the details of our new home. I plugged in the iPod and music blasted from the new speakers mounted in the ceiling. I turned up the volume so that the entire 1,200 square feet of our home was bathed with the opening strains of "Cielito Lindo" by Los Lobos. I didn't have to worry about disturbing upstairs or downstairs neighbors anymore. Morning sunlight streamed through the living room, casting a glow on the freshly painted gray walls. We had raised the ceiling by two feet but hadn't increased the square footage in the room. I marveled at the feeling of spaciousness those two feet lent the room; there was more air, more light, more warmth.

Everything felt new and clean. A walk-in shower with a teak bench and an array of nozzles made assisting Perry in the shower a cinch. Wide counter spaces in the bathroom let me move around him with ease when helping him shave. The den was enlarged to become our master bedroom with cork flooring, an upward-slanted ceiling, clerestory windows, and a walk-in closet. Light-blue glass tiles glistened in the expanded shower and tub in the guest bathroom. New skylights brightened the hallway that I lined with family photos.

I smiled as I moved from the living room toward the dining room, gliding on the hardwood floors in my socks. The pine floors were lighter now that they had been sanded and polished, and the removal of the entryway closet opened up the space between the dining room and living room. It didn't feel like the same cramped living room where Zack had built his sprawling LEGO structures or Paul did his monkey dance. Perry sat at the head of the dining room table, eating his bowl of cereal and fruit.

"Do you remember this song, Perry?" I asked.

He smiled.

"'Cielito Lindo'? Remember when we went to La Quinta for my birthday?"

He nodded yes.

"Remember when you asked the mariachis to play this song?"

He laughed out loud, nodded again, then closed his eyes. I could picture the scene from La Quinta fourteen years ago in vivid colors: the crisp blue skies with the Santa Rosa Mountains looming in the background, the desert heat beginning to rise from the expansive green lawns, the palm trees and riot of color in the pansies, impatiens, and marigolds that lined the grounds of the resort. It was my 40th birthday, the weekend after Thanksgiving, and we were enjoying Sunday brunch. We had just made our rounds of the sumptuous buffet, piling our plates with made-to-order omelets, carved roast beef, and hash browns. Perry tipped the serenading mariachis to sing "Happy Birthday." After they were done, the lead mariachi asked, "Any other requests?" Flustered, Perry blurted, "Cielito Lindo," a song he remembered from the old Frito Bandito commercials.

We had come to La Quinta after Perry and I spent a weekend there for his law firm's retreat and wanted to share the beauty of the resort with our boys. We played tennis on the regular courts, then the clay courts, then the grass courts. We soaked in the hot tub, staring up at the black desert night filled with stars, which we never saw from our house in Los Angeles. Wrapped in fluffy robes, we ordered room service and ate in the private enclosed courtyard to our casita. We frolicked in the pool. Perry did his imitation of a whale, jumping up and then slamming his full body back into the water with a big splash, while the boys squealed in the background.

It was a magical period in our lives, when eleven-year-old Zack and eight-year-old Paul were still happy to vacation with their parents, before they would transform into glum adolescents who would rather spend time with their friends. It was before I would go back to work full-time and feel torn about devoting energy to my career versus the family, before our lives would be upended by Perry's brain injury.

I looked back at Perry at the dining room table. His eyes were still closed, but his head was swaying to the music, a faint smile on his face.

"Ay, ay, ay, ay
Canta y no llores,
Sing and don't cry
Porque cantando se alegran,
Because singing gladdens
Cielito lindo, los corazones.
Pretty little heaven, one's heart."

Two or three years ago, the melody of this song and the memory of La Quinta would have stung my eyes with tears and engulfed me in sorrow for what was lost. But now I could listen to "Cielito Lindo" and remember the feeling of contentment at La Quinta and know that those hours of playing tennis and clowning in the pool laid the foundation for the caring and tenderness I would see in Zack and Paul as they tended to Perry. I felt reconciled with our new life. I could sit in my office downtown and gaze at the Gas Company tower where Perry's law firm was housed, and not feel pangs of sorrow. I could finger Perry's gray and navy business suits and feel okay about storing them in the back of the closet, knowing they represented another life. Like our newly remodeled home, I had gutted the remnants of our old lives and built a new one. I was no longer filled with sorrow or a longing to go back. The memory was enough.

CHAPTER 36

⁓⁝⁓

"I think you need to do something about the boat," said Manny on the phone. "I was down at the marina and the canvas cover is torn and shredded. The boat's being exposed to the elements."

I felt a pit in my stomach. I was in the middle of unpacking boxes. Moments earlier, I had been marveling at the amount of storage space in the maple cabinets in the new bathroom. Manny's phone call from across the street brought me back to earth. I didn't want to hear this. I had been avoiding Perry's fishing boat for the last six years because it was still too painful to deal with. It was dry docked in Marina del Rey. During our time in the marina, we didn't drive over to Mindanao Way once to visit it, even though Perry and I took long walks along all the other fingers of the marina, admiring the yachts and schooners we passed. The boat was too close to Perry's heart, my heart. It was the last vestige of his old life. I knew how much he had loved that boat.

We had bought it when Zack was eleven and Paul was nine. The boys had gone to sleep-away camp together that summer and for the first time since having children, Perry and I had five whole days alone together. I had envisioned romantic evenings at intimate restaurants, or going to plays or movies.

Perry had other plans. "After we drop the boys off in Long Beach, let's go to San Diego," he said. "I want to look for a fishing boat. Wouldn't it be great to have our own fishing boat? We could go out anytime we want."

Perry had gone out with fishing guides several times out of Redondo Beach and always came back exhilarated. *It would be nice for him to have his own boat,* I thought. It wasn't exactly what I had in mind for a romantic five days alone together but I went with him anyway to look at boats.

Near the end of the summer, Perry settled on a beige, 19-foot Key West fishing boat with a Johnson outboard motor and waist high chrome railings so he could fly fish in the ocean. He kept the name, 'Flytime,' because he read that you needed to properly christen a boat if you wanted to change its name. His eyes danced and his face radiated delight when he talked about Flytime. Slips were hard to rent in Marina del Rey so he found a dry dock that would hoist the boat into the water whenever he wanted.

"Come out on the boat with me," he pleaded. The first time I went, I got seasick. The next time I took Dramamine and spent the entire time in a groggy haze, dozing on the cushions in the bow. I hated the bumping on the waves and the loud drone of the engine. Paul loved being on Flytime. He would plant himself at the bow, taking on the wind and waves by hanging on to the railing. Zack joined them on occasion but decided he wasn't much of a fisherman.

We fell into a pattern after buying Flytime. At least once a month, Perry and Paul would wake at 6 a.m. and go north to Paradise Cove near Malibu or south near Palos Verdes. Most times, Manny accompanied them.

The first two years after we bought the boat, it didn't bother me that Perry and Paul went out once a month on weekend mornings, then napped the rest of the afternoon. I was still a stay-at-home mom. I had taken time off from work because I wanted to be there when they uttered their first word or when they learned to swim. Perry was supportive of my decision to stay home, even though he felt an increased weight and responsibility for the family.

"I feel like you can just tie a yoke on me and pull," he said one morning, as he got dressed for work. The boys and I were planning a "backwards" day where we did everything in reverse order. We would read in bed when they first woke up, then have dinner in the morning and eat breakfast at night. "You guys can just stay home and have fun," he said, a wistful tone in his voice as he knotted his tie.

His comment made me realize how fortunate I was to have the choice to stay home. For the next five years I catered to the needs of the boys and to Perry when he got home from work. I had never envisioned that I would grow up to be a housewife whose main responsibility was to make sure the household ran smoothly, but I enjoyed it.

Still, a part of me seemed to be missing. I loved being with the boys but I craved analytical work. I missed being among adults, puzzling over problems. Perry was excited when I decided to go back to graduate school to fulfill my dream of getting my Ph.D. Being in school was not as demanding as working a nine-to-five job. I attended classes when the boys were in school and studied at night after they went to bed. I could still attend Little League games and volunteer at their school. When Perry bought his boat, I was working on my dissertation and had the luxury of grocery shopping during the week, or running errands after I dropped the boys off at school so that my weekends were free.

Before I finished my dissertation, I received a job offer from a school reform organization and they were willing to let me work three quarter time so I could attend Zack and Paul's Little League games. Perry urged me to take it. "It will be a good way to ease back into the work world," he said.

But my return to work changed our comfortable home routine, especially after I finished my dissertation. The weekend hours became more precious. I resented the hours Perry spent on the boat and his long Saturday afternoons napping while I grocery shopped and ran errands.

During the week, Perry always wanted to have lunch together since we were both working downtown. But I was conscious of my shortened work hours, devoting an hour to lunch meant I had to work longer to finish my tasks, which was another hour taken away from the boys.

"Why won't you have lunch with me?" Perry asked. "You are always so busy, you don't have time for me."

"I do want to spend time with you," I said. "But you are always fishing on the weekends."

I was juggling work, home chores and chauffeuring the boys. But I knew his days were full and overflowing, too. He worked ten hour days at a frenetic pace at his law firm. Fishing on his boat was a balm for him, away from the creditors and debtors in his bankruptcy practice, away from e-mail, phones and faxes. But still, with my return to work, nothing in his life changed whereas everything in my life had. I was carrying the burden for the household. Each moment he spent on the boat was a moment away from me, from our family life and the never-ending home chores.

"We need to work this out," he said. "Have lunch with me."

I could detect the urgency in his voice. I agreed on Super Torta, tucked in a strip shopping mall where you could order and finish lunch in less than an hour. We ate our rib eye tortas in silence on the worn, purple chairs and Formica table. Beads of sweat formed on Perry's forehead as he ate, his tie tucked into the buttons of his white pressed shirt.

"Cyn, I don't want us to go on this way. You're angry all the time. I love you too much. I don't want this to go on and lead to divorce." Tears welled in his eyes. Perry never cried, he was always stoic. He looked miserable.

I put down my torta. "I don't either," I told him, feeling just as miserable. "We are mad at each other all the time. We used to have so much fun together. We need to listen to each other.

We need to find a happy medium."

Something shifted between us after that lunch at Super Torta. He listened to my complaints about household chores and needing help from him. I listened to him, without anger or jealousy, about how important fishing was to him. We made a vow to carve out time for each other. On weekends, he still went fishing but we shouldered the home duties together. He went to the grocery store with me, I went to the hardware store with him. I drove with him to Bob Marriott's Fly Fishing store and he browsed in Barnes and Noble with me. We both drove the boys to their hockey games, or picked them up from friend's houses.

As we sat together in the car waiting for the boys or in the stands at their hockey games, our easy banter returned. We recited grocery lists, puzzled through work issues, gossiped about acquaintances, reminisced about our college days, fantasized about future travel plans, or what we would do when the boys went off to college, or how we would spend our days in retirement. Even the most mundane tasks were more fun when we were together.

He even convinced me to go out on the boat with him. "There's a run of white sea bass in Santa Monica Bay. These fish are huge, you can get a 50 pounder," he said. "Come with me!"

All four of us went on the boat that weekend, leaving at 9 a.m. instead of 6 a.m. I took my Dramamine and braced myself while the boat powered out to sea, a cold mist spraying as we slammed against the waves. Five miles out, Perry cut the engine and Paul put in the anchor. Dense fog reduced our visibility to less than ten feet in each direction. I curled up on the cushions at the bow, wrapped my fleece jacket tightly around me. The bobbing and swaying of the boat lulled me into a half sleep. Perry and Paul cast out and waited. And waited. When I woke an hour later, I asked, "How much longer?"

"Just twenty more minutes and we'll leave," said Perry. By then, Paul was dozing, too. I settled back down on the cushions. Then we heard Perry yell, "I got one!"

Paul was up in a flash, gaffe hook in one hand, the net in the other. Zack hovered nearby. Perry hauled in his line, the reel zinging. Then there it was, a giant white sea bass, 48 inches long. It was the biggest fish I had ever seen him haul out of Santa Monica Bay. Paul tried to weigh it on the boga grip but it was over 40 pounds. Fisherman in a boat twenty feet away came closer for a view. "It's a beaut!" they hollered. Perry beamed when the boys took turns with him posing with the giant fish on the dock when we returned to the marina.

Later that night, Perry cupped my face in his hands and kissed me. "That was the best day ever, because you were there with me."

FLYTIME HAD SAT IDLE FOR six years now. The first year after his heart attack, we took it out in the marina. Perry caressed the hull when he first saw the boat but once in the water, it was up to Paul to start up the engine, maneuver it out of the slip and through the channels. We motored in the marina only, keeping the no-wake speed of eight knots. We didn't feel emboldened enough to go past the breakwater to open sea. Perry sat in the bow smiling but gave no indication he knew how to steer the boat, work the knots on the cleats, manage the bumpers or lift the skag on the motor. He stared at his fishing poles and reels with a blank expression. It was too painful to watch.

And yet, I could not face giving up this boat that was so dear to Perry's heart. I knew I couldn't summon the energy to learn how to start the engine or steer it into the slip, much less take it out into the open ocean. For several years I put out feelers for someone to take him out on his boat but never found anyone who was experienced with boating and brain injury.

I could see the distress on Paul's face when I asked if he wanted to take his father out. Paul's interest in fishing died after the brain injury, and the boat was a constant reminder of the special time they spent together. Manny gave up fishing entirely for two years after Perry's heart attack. For all of us, letting go of this boat meant that we were giving up somehow, acknowledging that Perry would never come back.

"If Paul is free this Saturday," Manny said, "I can help him clean out the boat. We'll wash out all the dirt, get new tarps for it."

I inhaled a deep breath. I knew this was Manny's way of telling me it was time to let go. I slowly exhaled and found my voice again. The last vestige of the old Perry was becoming untethered, ready to drift away.

"Okay," I said, "Thank you, Manny."

LATER THAT YEAR, AFTER PAUL and Manny cleaned out the dirt and fixed a new tarp over the top, my brother-in-law Ernie offered to help us sell the boat. He drove his truck from Salinas so he could hitch up the boat and trailer to drive back to central California. He had thought of everything: spare tires for the trailer in case they were flat, extra wires to hook up brake lights and blinkers, even a license plate with a current registration sticker because I couldn't find ours. I choked back tears as he drove out of the dock parking lot but Perry stood unfazed, watching silently.

A few weeks later, I felt relieved and grateful when my nephew reported that they sold the boat to a young man in his 20s who loved to fish.

Flytime had a new home.

CHAPTER 37

⸻

It had seemed like such an easy thing when we first considered buying a vacation home in Mammoth. Zack was the one who put the idea in my head. "Start envisioning a life after you stop working," he suggested, after I lamented that eight years after Perry's brain injury, my daily life consisted of working long hours and then caregiving at home. "It's time to think of a transition strategy from work," he said.

A home in the mountains is what I started to envision. We had always loved the eastern Sierra, and after Perry's brain injury we continued to visit Mammoth every summer, opting for the convenience of rented condominiums and taking day hikes. Perry loved the mountain air, and each year I felt wistful when we left, knowing that a long weekend once a year was not enough time to enjoy the outdoors.

If we had our own place in Mammoth, we could take many more long weekends out of town, and when I retired we could spend weeks or months in the mountains. I pictured us drifting on a rowboat on Lake George in the summer, watching the aspen trees turn orange and gold in the fall, or sitting by a wood-burning stove while snow covered the mountains in winter. I thought of how much easier caregiving would be in a place that we owned. We could outfit the shower with handheld nozzles, grab bars, and a shower bench. I wouldn't have to worry if the stairs were too steep for him or what the configurations of rooms were whenever we rented a condo.

I felt a spark of excitement as I combed through real estate listings on the Internet, studying pictures of living rooms, bathrooms, and kitchens. The timing was right: after graduating from Bowdoin, Paul committed to spending another season as a forest ranger and was looking for a place to live in Mammoth. Interest rates were at an all-time low and property prices had dropped into an affordable range. We enlisted a broker and found a three-bedroom, two-bathroom place with a wood-burning stove, hardwood floors, and high ceilings. The unit could accommodate Perry's needs also, with an attached bathroom to the master bedroom and wide stairs.

The real estate process flowed seamlessly. As I started the loan process, I explained to the bank officer that my husband was brain injured, and I wanted to know the easiest way to apply for the loan and take title. I didn't want to subject Perry to the hundreds of documents he would need to sign. The bank officer was unfazed.

"Can he write his signature?" she asked.

"Yes," I said.

"It's up to you. When we close, he will have to sign and initial all the documents, which are pages and pages. If you don't think he can sign all those documents, you can take the loan and title out in your name only, and then he would only need to sign a quit claim deed and get it notarized," she said. "If you take the loan out with both your names, the bank is going to have to verify his disability income, and they'll want to know whether it's a permanent disability. They will probably ask for a doctor's statement and a letter from the insurance company."

I squirmed. Did I need to drag all of his medical information into this process? It seemed so invasive. We had enough assets to cover the loan anyway. What right did they have to pry into all this information about the nature of his disability? Since I qualified for a loan based on my income, I took the path of least resistance and took title in my name only. The last step to owning a condo in Mammoth was to have Perry sign the quit claim deed and get it notarized.

I KNEW HE WAS TROUBLE as soon as he started up the front steps. It wasn't the pompadour hair style or the frayed leather jacket or the white shirt unbuttoned to reveal a hairy chest. It was the way he chewed his gum, open-mouthed and nervous, like a teenage girl. When he extended his hand to shake mine, I detected a New Jersey accent in his "How ya doing?"

I was already annoyed that he was twenty minutes late. I had rushed home from work to be on time because he insisted on the phone that he could do 7:00 but not 7:30. He called at 7:20 to say, "I can't find your house. I'm in front of 3389 but I can't find 3385."

"It's next door to your right. We are the next house over to 3389," I replied. Maybe it was hard to read house numbers in the dark.

"Oh, I guess the numbers go down instead of up," he said.

I opened the front door to find him standing in my neighbor's driveway.

He stepped into the house, looked around the living room, and said, "You gotta nice place here." Under the living room lights, I could see flecks of gray in his brown hair and the wrinkles on his tanned, leathery skin. In his left ear two small, silver hoops glistened.

"Now, let me get settled here," he said, still chomping on his gum as I guided him to the kitchen table. He sat down and placed his carrier bag on his lap, took out his notary ledger, his stamp, a ruler, two pens, and the inkpad for the thumbprint.

"Whatta we signing here?" he asked.

"It's a quit claim deed," I said.

He looked through the document, then faced Perry. "Do

you know what you are signing?" he asked. Perry nodded yes. The man opened his ledger and drew lines across the page with his ruler, then slowly printed Perry's name, address, driver's license number. He handed the quit claim deed to Perry.

"Okay, sign right here," he said.

Perry signed his name on the document, but the end of his signature trailed off the dotted line.

"Wait, that signature doesn't match his driver's license," the notary said, his chewing more vigorous now. Even before Perry's brain injury, his signature was illegible; he formed the P in his first name and L in his last name, but the rest was a squiggly line. Since the brain injury his handwriting had gotten smaller and less firm on the page, but he still formed the P and L in the same manner. But this was not passing muster with the notary.

"He had a heart attack," I said. I wasn't going to say anything about his brain injury. "His signature is the same, though." I looked at Perry's picture from his driver's license, taken well before his heart attack, his somber face and chubby cheeks, free of brain injury, in a suit and tie. He looked skinnier now and his face was even more serious, but it was clearly him.

"I don't know," said the notary, still staring at the driver's license. "Let's see how he signs in here," pushing the ledger book toward Perry. "He has to sign on a straight line."

I thought of all the times we had documents notarized. No one had ever said that the signature had to be on a straight line. Perry signed the ledger book with a firmer, straighter signature. But the notary was not satisfied.

"Does he know what he's signing? Does he have the capacity to sign this?" He turned to Perry. "What's today's date?"

Perry looked at him with a blank stare.

"He had a heart attack, and he doesn't have short-term memory," I told him. "He doesn't remember the day of the week."

I knew then I had made a big mistake. What was I thinking, calling a notary from the Internet to sign this document?

Of course he would question this transaction. He had no knowledge of our context, our lives. I could be a charlatan trying to trick Perry into transferring title to me. How was this notary, who couldn't even find our address on this small street, to know?

"He doesn't know today's date!" said the notary, looking at Perry and then at me. "He doesn't know what he is signing! He's not competent!"

I stared at the notary, at the silver rings on his fingers clutching the quit claim deed, which Perry had just signed. *Just sign and stamp the damn thing*, I wanted to shout. I was fully aware of Perry's deficits. I had spent the last eight years living it day to day, constantly aware of what it's like to live with someone who never remembered he was disabled, could not fend for himself, and was not capable of expressing what he knew. I had worked hard to stitch together a network of support where the line between ability and disability blurred. Our friends and family didn't treat him as if he was incompetent; they conversed and joked with him as they always did. I made sure we maintained his dignity and respect and did not treat him as if he was lacking or less than. I felt my cheeks flare with hot anger.

"I don't feel comfortable notarizing this," he said. "He doesn't even know what day it is."

Was it his place to question Perry's capacity? I thought he was supposed to affirm that Perry was the person signing the document. Did this notary have training in neuropsychology? Could this entire real estate transaction become undone because of this notary? The bank officer didn't mention anything about capacity or competency. She just wanted a signed, notarized document.

"Forget it," I said, standing up from the table. "If you don't feel comfortable notarizing this, then don't."

"You shouldda told me this before. I'm sorry, I can't do this. I'm gonna tear up this quit claim deed and take it with me."

He stood up and tore up the document. It was my only

copy.

"I don't need to have this discussion with you," I said as I walked to the front door and opened it. "You can just leave now."

"You know, you're not going to find another notary that's going to sign this for you. I'm sorry."

I slammed the front door after he left. When the anger subsided I was filled with cold fear. What were my alternatives now? I could put Perry on the loan and title, but there were ten times as many documents that he would have to sign and notarize. Wouldn't a notary raise the same issue about his capacity to sign loan and title documents? Maybe my only course of action was to go to court and have him declared incompetent and become his conservator. We had dealt with this issue eight years ago, shortly after his brain injury, but the attorney didn't recommend it. It wasn't just the court proceedings and reporting requirements that terrified me. It was the finality of the decision, the fact that Perry would be considered legally incompetent that scared me. I had kept it at bay and didn't want to face it.

Escrow was scheduled to close in the next week. Paul had already given notice at his apartment and was ready to move in to the condo. Would I have to delay everything for months while I went through court proceedings? I called Rich, Perry's former law partner, for advice.

"This isn't my area of expertise, but I'm sure we can find a solution. I'll consult with the head of our real estate group at the firm tomorrow to get their best thinking," he said. "How about calling your estate attorneys? They are used to dealing with issues of conservatorship and signatures. Maybe they can help."

My dreams that night were filled with anxious worry. For the past eight years, I had worked so hard to focus our lives on ability, rather than disability, to concentrate on what we could do in spite of his brain injury, rather than what we couldn't do because of his deficits. The boys and I looked for ways to accommodate Perry's disability, rather than give in to it. It was the only way I could keep moving forward with hope and optimism. Otherwise I could sink into a sea of sadness and sorrow at what was taken away. This vacation home meant that we could make the wilderness a regular part of our routine again, that we could rebuild a semblance of our former lives. But was it now out of grasp because my husband was brain damaged? I felt myself sinking, submerged in disability.

IN THE MORNING I CALLED Emily, our estate attorney, and spilled out my worries about getting the document notarized, Perry's capacity, and whether I should file for conservatorship. In less than a minute, she pulled up our files on her computer.

"First of all, it sounds like you got a bad notary. It's not their job to question capacity. They are supposed to authenticate the signature and verify that the person signing the form is indeed him."

Her soft, calming voice was an elixir for my nerves. My tension eased as I heard her tapping on her keyboard, scanning through our files.

"Theoretically Perry doesn't even need to sign a quit claim deed because you have power of attorney for him. You can sign all legal documents for him. We set that up for you when we established your community property trust, remember?"

I remembered the thick binder they had sent us with trust documents, wills, health directives, and power of attorney forms. I had focused on moving our assets into the community property trust and didn't read through the rest of the binder.

"Even if you did put the loan and title in both names, you could sign on his behalf. He doesn't need to sign anything," she said. "Why don't you call the bank and see if you can just sign the quit claim deed for him? If not, just bring Perry in and we can have him sign and notarize the form. Notaries are very nervous now because of the whole financial fiasco. A lot of them have had to go to court because they were doing 'roto-notaries' during the mortgage mess. That's probably why the notary was so skittish."

"But what about conservatorship?" I asked. "Should I move with those proceedings?"

"You already have full power of attorney for him," she said. "That means you can act on his behalf for all real estate and financial transactions, insurance, annuity, litigation, just about everything. Is there anyone questioning or contesting your care? Are you having problems with doctors or medical care?"

"No." In the years post brain injury, I had battled to get him the care he needed, but no one questioned my right to advocate on his behalf, and no one had challenged my handling of finances.

"Then you are fine. Conservatorship is a very onerous process, and one of the first things the court asks is why a power of attorney doesn't suffice."

A sense of relief washed over me. I wanted to reach through the phone lines and give Emily a kiss and a hug. I should have called her first before starting this real estate transaction. I could feel the threads of my safety net weaving together and tightening again, returning me to the world of ability.

Within two weeks, the condo was ours.

CHAPTER 38

―᠈ᴗᴗᴗ―

"Go back to sleep," I hissed at Perry. It was 2:00 in the morning and we were in our newly purchased condo in Mammoth, sleeping in twin beds in the only room that was habitable. The other two bedrooms downstairs were still in the process of being painted, and were bare of furniture. Disoriented, he kept waking, sitting up and walking to my bed, trying to climb in. He wasn't used to us sleeping in separate beds and he was in a foreign environment. But at 2:00 in the morning, I didn't care. My body ached from cleaning and unpacking the condo and I had been immersed in deep sleep. I threw off my covers and stood up, then guided him back to his own bed.

"This is your bed," I said, pushing him down and tucking his legs under the blankets. "Go to sleep." I climbed back to my own bed. I heard the squeaking of his mattress, the rustling of sheets as he moved about, turning onto his left side, then his right side. I had already taken him to the bathroom so I knew he wasn't wet. Maybe he was uncomfortable from the polyester in the cheap blankets, which were making me sweat. I had bought the comforter and quilt covers on sale and didn't notice that they weren't 100% cotton. I waited for the moving to stop, closed my eyes and tried to remember my interrupted dream.

Ten minutes later, as I felt my body being lulled into sleep, I heard the polyester quilt fall to the floor. I opened my eyes and could see in the semi-darkness that Perry was sitting up again. He saw me turn my head and stood, reaching towards me. I threw back my blankets again and pushed him onto his bed, this time not as gently as the first.

"No," I said, through clenched teeth. "This is your bed. You have to sleep in this bed. Now lie down and go to sleep." I held him down and considered pinning him down but how? I tossed the blankets back on top of him, not caring if they were straight and tucked in.

I moved back to my bed and pulled the covers over me, then stared at the wooden beams in the ceiling, visible from the moonlight through the window shades. Since his brain injury, he had these bouts of restlessness every three or four months. He would wake in the middle of the night and even after I took him to the bathroom to change a wet diaper or the bed pad or the sheets, he would still be awake, tossing and turning, sitting up, searching for something that he could not verbalize and I could not discern. It was during those dark hours in the middle of the night, when I was half-conscious, half in a dream-like state that I felt the edges of insanity.

"What is wrong with you?" I would yell, knowing that he couldn't rationally explain what he needed. "Why won't you sleep, why won't you let me sleep?"

I knew from all the brochures and caregiver guides given to me by the rehabilitation specialists that I shouldn't raise my voice and get angry, that I should speak in calming tones and redirect him to bed and not use force. But at 2:00 or 4:00 in the morning, rationality vanished and I longed for restraints to tie him down. I yelled, I pleaded, "Go back to sleep! If you don't go back to sleep, I will put you in a nursing home!" I would be thinking about the alarm going off at 6:15, the 45 minute commute downtown and the full day of meetings that awaited me at work. At the mention of a nursing home, he always looked at me in confusion with a hardness in his expression that in pre-brain injury days meant he was ready to argue back. But in his brain injured state, he didn't say anything in response. I could only detect the sense of hurt and betrayal in his face.

The neurologist prescribed a sedative, Clonazepam, for these sleepless nights but I used it sparingly. We had worked so hard to get him to wake from his coma and to get his brain stimulated that I hated to sedate him. But on those restless nights, I gave in and doled out half the dosage, afraid that he would fall into a catatonic stupor again. If the agitation persisted, I would escape to the twin bed in the boys' room, empty since they had left for college. I would stare at the ceiling and wonder, *Why me? Why us? What have we done in this life to deserve this?* I thought about one of my girlfriends, a woman whom I had known since our oldest son Zack started preschool fifteen years ago.

"I always thought something like this would happen to my husband because he has such an unhealthy lifestyle," she had said to me, after hearing about Perry's heart attack. "He never exercises and he's overweight. I wonder how my kids would react if this happened to my husband," she said. "They don't have the close relationship that Zack and Paul do with Perry. I don't know if they would be as kind as Zack and Paul."

So why did this happen to my husband instead of hers? In those moments, I hated his brain injury, hated my fate. I wondered how much longer I would have to do this and what will happen when we grow old and I can't tend to him anymore. Could I put him in a nursing home and have someone else deal with him?

I imagined what my life would be like with him in a nursing home and of the freedom I would have from caregiving. I could travel, I could attend conferences without having to make accommodations for early flights and caregivers. I could go to shopping malls and browse bookstores without worrying about him losing his balance or having to walk too far or squeezing my hand so tightly that it hurt. I could pop into a store for a quick errand, jog on the beach or ride my bike.

On those nights when he didn't sleep, when he was overcome by restlessness, it was pure hell. I hated waking up in the middle of the night and trying to talk sense to him, knowing he was not comprehending and was beyond reasoning. Was this better than not having him at all?

After the third time Perry stood up that night in Mammoth, I gave him half a sedative and waited for him to settle into sleep. But his restlessness continued. This time, there was no other room to escape to. Paul was sleeping on the couch in the living room and the downstairs rooms had no furniture or heat. I stared at the wooden beams in the ceiling, feeling the knot in my back that no massage could ease. How many times have I had to endure these night terrors, when restlessness and agitation made me the crazy one?

Somehow I had imagined that life would be easier in our own vacation home. But buying a vacation home did not change any of this. We could own three homes, five homes, but this part of my life would never change. Perry will always be brain injured, he will have these bouts of agitation, he will have restless nights whether we are home in Los Angeles or in our vacation condo in Mammoth. Maybe it was time to look into placing him in a nursing home.

I heard the movement of blankets again. He stood up. I sighed. I turned on the light and moved to his bed. His face was masked in confusion and he looked at me with questioning eyes. I took a different tack. I gently guided him back into his bed, looked into his eyes and whispered in a calm voice.

"These are single beds. There is no room for the two of us. You have to sleep here and I will be right across the room from you in the other bed. When we go home, we will have our bigger bed and we can sleep together again. Do you understand?"

He nodded yes and his eyes softened in comprehension, then closed. I straightened out the covers, then turned out the light, and crawled back into my bed. He slept through the rest of the night.

In the morning, sunlight streamed through the shades and the room was bathed in soft yellow. Outside, the cloudless sky was deep blue and a light dusting of snow covered the ground. Everything looked clean and fresh, the darkness and desperation in the middle of the night forgotten. I looked at Perry, still in deep sleep on his back. In repose, his face was relaxed, the soft inhale and exhale of his breathing visible in his chest. I walked to his bed and studied his pink cheeks and the stubble of his beard. In the light, he looked so normal, so unmarred by brain injury. I regretted my thoughts about putting him in a nursing home. How could I conceive of abandoning him in that way? Would they care for him the way I do, would they carefully shave his chin, and comb his tufts of hair to the right? Would they gaze in the mirror with him after his morning routine and tell him he looks handsome? I reached down and kissed his cheek. He opened his eyes and his face lit up at the sight of me and there was his smile, the one that captivated me at age eighteen and appeared every time he saw me. He held my hand to his lips and gently kissed it.

"Good morning, Perry," I said.

The idea of placing Perry in a nursing home came up again months later when I met Sandy for drinks after work. The same thing had happened to her husband: cardiac arrest, lack of oxygen and a resulting anoxic brain injury. We had connected through a support group of women with brain injured husbands and exchanged emails. I sent her a link to an essay I wrote about caregiving. "We have got to meet!" she wrote back. "Your story is my story!"

We agreed to meet for drinks at Roy's downtown since she worked nearby. I didn't know what she looked like but knew it was her when I spotted a woman with frosted blonde hair swept in a bun and a fitted brown pant suit. I felt an instant connection when her brown eyes twinkled as she extended her hand, then dropped it and reached to give me a hug instead. Like mine, her husband had owned a boat and loved the wilderness. Sandy had researched the same rehabilitation programs and community resources I had and discovered the same result—there was not much out there for brain injured patients. I felt as if we had been friends forever, sharing intimacies that only those who had been through the same ordeal can. There was no judgment, no horror at the details of caregiving, no shock or awe. We had lived through the same hell.

Her husband didn't seem as disabled as Perry. He wasn't incontinent and he was much more verbal but he had suffered more frontal lobe damage and was prone to mood swings and angry outbursts. When he was discharged from the rehabilitation center, Sandy struggled to keep him home but his behavior was unpredictable. He had threatened her and her adult daughter with violence, he shouted at inappropriate times. She made the decision to place him in a residential facility 90 minutes from Los Angeles.

"It was either him or me," she said. "I was going down with the ship. I was on medication for depression, I went to therapy, I couldn't eat, I couldn't sleep. Everyone kept telling me I had to place him somewhere to save myself." As she twisted the cocktail napkin in her hands, I could see the underlying sadness in her eyes. She was haunted by guilt for placing him in a facility, but I couldn't blame her. If Perry had exhibited the same type of behavior as Sandy's husband, I probably would have put him in a facility, too.

"You are doing the right thing," I said to Sandy. "No one can tell you what you feel is right or wrong. You are doing the best you can for him."

"There are times when I wished he didn't survive the cardiac arrest," she said. "I wonder if he or we would be better off if he hadn't."

Her voice trailed off and I nodded.

"Yes, I have thought that myself hundreds of times," I said.

"You should come out to residential facility with me some weekend. My husband really likes it there. He's not angry or agitated when he's there. He loves the outdoors and they have these spacious lawns and it's away from the city. It's like being in the wilderness. You should just come and see it. You never know what will happen with Perry."

I felt wistful when we parted that evening, and a bit envious of Sandy's freedom. She wouldn't have to fix dinner for her husband when she got home or take him to the bathroom, or worry about being home in time to relieve the caregiver. She could stop a store any time she wanted and not have to deal with helping her husband in and out of the car or guiding him when he walked so that he didn't lose his balance. But her burdens were just as heavy as mine in terms of being responsible for the care of her husband.

SANDY'S IDEA OF VISITING THE residential facility lodged in my mind. Should I go visit? Could I conceive of placing Perry there? All through his rehabilitation, we had been adverse to any placement hinting at a nursing home, we just wanted him home. But would the day come when I could not physically or mentally care for him anymore?

I talked it over with the boys. "Dad doesn't seem to be uncontrollable at home, does he?" said Paul. "I mean, you are still able to take care of him, right?"

"Well, there are those moments when I get overwhelmed," I said, recalling the nights when he was restless and I faced a day of meetings ahead of me and I slept in the spare bedroom.

"I still think the good outweighs the bad in having him at home. You are still able to travel and do what you like even though he's not in a home. It doesn't seem like the burden is unbearable. I'd say keep it in mind as a backup for when you do feel like it's unbearable."

I called Zack to get his perspective. "I don't know about

putting him in a home. You've got a pretty good deal right now. Arnold has been Dad's caregiver for over six years now and you trust him. What do you know about the people in this facility? Plus, you seem to be managing it all pretty well, you have Manny and Nancy across the street to help out. I'd say give it serious thought if you feel like you can't endure this anymore."

Was I brave enough to live in our home alone, without Perry? I had never lived alone. I had gone from my childhood home straight to college to live with roommates and then lived with Perry since then. As a child, I suffered from insomnia when my oldest sister got married when I was twelve and I had my own room for the first time. Even now as an adult, I didn't fall asleep easily when I was alone. When I traveled by myself, I kept a light on in my hotel room. I found comfort in Perry's presence on those nights when he wasn't restless and I slept peacefully listening to his deep breaths and soft snores. I wondered how I would fare sleeping alone in our house or in our condo in Mammoth. Would I lie awake, alarmed by the creaks and groans of the house, scared by the patter of raccoons as they moved across the roof? Would I be plagued by the insomnia of my youth all over again?

Even in his disabled state, I felt safer when he was with me. His presence grounded me. On Sunday nights, when I took the last bag of trash out to the garbage can on the curb late at night, he would stand in the doorway, looking after me because he knew I got spooked by walking out into the dark street. I thought of all the times we drove to Mammoth after I got off work, hitting the road at 6 or 7 in the evening and arriving well after midnight at our condo. I didn't think I had the courage to do that on my own, even though driving with a brain injured husband probably made me more vulnerable than being alone. I thought about how much I would miss his daily presence if I put him in a homea nd the glow on his face when he saw me. I needed him as much as he needed me.

But the idea that I could put him in a home, that I had an

actual facility that would be good for him stayed with me. If it got to be too much, this was an escape hatch if I ever needed it. I carried that idea in my back pocket and thought about it on weekends, when after an exhausting week at work, all I wanted to do was sit on the couch and play games on my iPad but had to take Perry to the bathroom or urge him to drink water. I thought about it when his fingers and toes were cold, almost purple and I couldn't warm them up even though the cardiologist assured me his heart was pumping fine. I thought about it when I woke in the middle of the night and had to change wet sheets, then would lie awake for hours afterwards, unable to sleep. I thought about it in those moments when I felt like I couldn't endure caregiving any longer, when I thought, *this is it, this is how it feels to break, this is how my façade of bravado crumbles and I could become a catatonic zombie or a self-destructing alcoholic.* I would hold the idea of the facility in the back of my mind and say, *I don't have to put up with this. I could put him in the same facility as Sandy's husband.* And somehow, that would get me through the day or night, that would give me the strength to continue on the next day.

A FEW MONTHS AFTER I met Sandy, I got an email from her saying someone had "shoved" her husband at the residential facility and he fell, breaking his hip. He was now hospitalized and they would have to do surgery to repair his hip. My heart went out to her for having to face another incident, another calamity. A few weeks later, another email came. He came through the surgery okay but was heavily drugged, barely speaking and not responsive. He had regressed in terms of his brain injury recovery and was not speaking anymore. His spot at the residential facility was no longer available and the hospital wanted to put him in a nursing home. Sandy was back to square one, having to navigate the maze of health insurance, placements and rehabilitation facilities all over again.

"I'm so sorry," I wrote back. I felt let down too, for having thought that the residential facility would have been a good place for Perry. Now I knew I couldn't do it. I could not surrender his care to someone else no matter how wide the lawns or how nice the staff was. The weight of responsibility was all mine again. There was no escape hatch.

Chapter 39

For the past ten years, I faithfully paid Perry's dues of $125 to the State Bar of California to keep him in active status. But this year, ten years later, as I looked over the form, I wondered if I needed to keep the membership active. Perry was never going to be a lawyer again. He didn't remember what he did yesterday or an hour ago. He couldn't drive, he couldn't dress himself and he hardly spoke. Was I just deluding myself in keeping this membership alive? Was I just holding on to false hope, just like I did with his fishing boat before I gave that up? I had to face reality. He would never be able to practice law again.

It wasn't an outrageous amount of money but I thought about what I could have bought with $125. It would pay for half a day of caregiving or a speech therapy session. Multiplied over the years, it totaled $1,250, the cost of a month of physical therapy. Or it would have paid for several pairs of pants with elastic waists or sandals with Velcro ties for Perry. It would have paid for a facial or a massage for me. I decided to let the membership lapse.

A few months later, I received a notice that they were

assessing a $20 fine as a late fee. Apparently, it wasn't like a magazine subscription that you could just let lapse. You had to formally withdraw from the association and there were instructions on how to request resignation forms. I sighed. I called the number on the form and explained to the operator that my husband was brain injured and not capable of practicing law and wanted to withdraw from the bar association.

She hesitated. "Well, if he ever decides to practice law again or wants to go to active status, he will have to pay all the penalties."

"Yes, I understand," I said.

"Are you sure he wants to resign?" she asked. "If he resigns, he will have to reapply for the bar and take the exam again."

Now I was the one who hesitated. Take the bar again? I remembered how hard he had worked all through law school and the hours and days he spent studying for the bar after his graduation. We were living in Berkeley that summer and while he studied at the library late into the night, I made all our wedding arrangements and went out with friends. He had been so focused and intent on preparing for the bar that I admired his discipline and his ability to not get distracted by the wedding plans swirling around him. During the exam, his friend had rented a hotel room in San Francisco near the law school in case the BART broke down and he couldn't commute across the bay. He had suggested Perry do the same. But Perry had said he slept better at home next to me. During those nights of the three day exam, he was tense and restless and he woke with the sheets twisted around his body each morning. He had passed on his first try and I couldn't imagine him going through that ordeal again.

"Yes, I understand," I said to the woman on the phone. "Please send us the resignation forms."

A thick packet arrived in the mail several days later. Tucked in with the resignation form were instructions for filing a petition for reinstatement with the State Bar Court of California filling an entire page. There was also a four page document summarizing a hearing disposition of a lawyer who had resigned from the bar when he retired but now had a job opportunity to practice law again. He had not realized how "precious" his state bar membership was and was not aware of how difficult it would be to regain active status after resigning. He had to have ten witnesses attest to his moral standing and had to present evidence of his learning and ability to support his reinstatement, which was then deliberated and finally approved by the court.

I was intimidated by all the legal language. I should have listened to Rich, Perry's law firm partner, and just kept paying the membership. I remembered when months after his heart attack, his work colleagues had emptied out his corner office and delivered boxes of papers to our home. I had sorted through them and sat with Rich to see which memberships I needed to keep.

"You can forget about these," said Rich, as he went through the papers for Lexis/Nexis and the LA County Bar Association. "But you don't want this one to lapse," he said, holding the State Bar of California form. "This one is important."

Now I understood why. Even though he wasn't going to practice law again, I didn't want to have to go through this big deal by formally resigning, then having his case discussed at a hearing of the State Bar and being listed among attorneys that had been disbarred. I had to keep that last piece of his dignity.

Besides, what if some miracle happened and he did recover? What if, in the next ten years, there was a breakthrough in brain research and they discovered a stem cell that could restore lost brain cells? I had to hang on to that last thread of hope. I paid the fine and renewed his yearly membership.

CHAPTER 40

~\|/~

"What do you do for fun?" my friend Ellen asked me over dinner on one of the rare evenings I went out without Perry.

I was caught off guard. What did I do for fun? I sometimes took vacations without Perry or traveled on business by myself. Those occasions were always a welcome respite. When I thought of my day-to-day life, I wondered if I even had "fun" anymore. My life consisted of ten-hour days at work, then coming home to tend to Perry, taking him to the bathroom, urging him to take another bite of his dinner. My weekends were spent grocery shopping and on household errands that I couldn't get to during the week.

Other than work and caregiving, what was the shape of my life now? I wasn't a law firm wife anymore and our kids were no longer involved in activities where I met fellow parents. We didn't go to law firm functions and make chit chat over cocktails. After Zack and Paul moved out, we didn't go to sporting events, either. Many of our friends and acquaintances had fallen away, especially Perry's colleagues from his law firm. During their visits, I was the one that did all the talking for him but their connection had been with him, not me. Our social circle had gotten much smaller and our lives had turned inward as we spent more time at home. We didn't eat out as often at fancy restaurants and we didn't go to plays or concerts anymore, other than the Hollywood Bowl. We hadn't even visited the new Disney Hall downtown.

Our lives pre-brain injury had been full with social events, dinners out with friends, fundraisers, and sporting events. In all of those activities Perry and I had been one unit, always together. My sense of contentment had been dependent on Perry as my partner.

I remembered when Perry said to me, twenty years ago, "You can't depend on me for your happiness." He had just graduated from law school at UC Hastings in San Francisco and I had completed my master's in social work from UC Berkeley. It was the 1980s and President Reagan had just made massive cuts to social services. My job prospects in social work were bleak so we knew we should go wherever Perry got the best job, which happened to be a law firm in Los Angeles. I reluctantly agreed to the move. I had loved living in the Bay Area. I was near my mother and grandmother and I had a close group of friends from social work school. After our wedding, I had blinked back tears as I said goodbye to my mother and grandmother before we moved to Los Angeles. I hated to leave them.

"It's okay," said my grandmother, holding my hand, trying to comfort me. "It's just like in China when a woman marries and she goes to the husband's village. Just think of this like you are moving to Perry's village in Los Angeles."

But I hated the Los Angeles "village." I hated the traffic, I hated the fine layer of soot that settled on the windowsill of our apartment that faced a busy commuter street. I missed Moe's and Cody's bookstores, my family, my circle of friends. In L.A., I had transferred to the Westwood office of the Social Security Administration and interviewed claimants for disability. It was dull and menial most days. I felt like a faceless bureaucrat as

I interviewed homeless or mentally ill claimants and could do nothing except try to expedite the processing of their claims. Perry, on the other hand, had his own private office and was swept into bankruptcy practice with social cocktail hours after work and firm dinners at fancy restaurants. I envied his position at the law firm, his sense of purpose and accomplishment. I resented the long hours he worked as I escaped at 5:00 each day and sat at home, waiting for him to return.

That was when he said, "You can't depend on me for your happiness," as I complained about living in Los Angeles and the long hours he worked. "You need to find a social network, something that interests you."

I was incensed and hurt. I had just uprooted myself from Berkeley to follow him here. "What are you talking about?" I asked. "Don't you miss being together?"

"Of course, I do," he said. "I love spending time together. I'm not saying that I don't love you or don't want to spend time with you. I just think you need to find other interests and not be constantly waiting for me to come home from work."

His words stung. In Santa Barbara and Berkeley, I had an independent life from Perry, with my own interests. Somehow, in the move I had lost my sense of self and became a dependent, whiny and nagging wife.

I started to explore Los Angeles on my own, spending long hours at the Papa Bach Bookstore on Santa Monica Boulevard and at the Either/Or in Hermosa Beach. I rode my bike along San Vicente Boulevard to the beach, took Chinese brush painting and sign language classes and volunteered for an Adult Literacy program. By the time I switched jobs to work at the school district as a policy analyst a year later, I had a group of friends of my own and activities that stimulated me. I was beginning to enjoy the swaying palm trees, the jacaranda trees that bathed the street in purple petals and the expanse of sand and beach from the bluffs at Palisades Park. Over time, it dawned on me that I wasn't dependent on Perry for my own happiness. I had redeveloped an identity that was mine alone and not part of a couple.

With the onset of parenthood and active careers, it was hard to maintain independent activities that didn't include Perry or the boys. Now, after his brain injury, I wondered if his words back then were a harbinger of things to come. Did he somehow know that I would have to rely on my own sense of self and not on him to keep me happy? I wasn't dependent on him anymore for my source of happiness. I was content to stay home and at peace with the quietness that encompassed our home. I didn't miss cocktail chatter, concerts and baseball games. I wasn't filled with woe and pity. Although my well of sorrow was still present from time to time, it had faded to become a part of the backdrop of our present life, like a dull noise in the ether.

Perry's brain injury had not made him aggressive or angry. In his passivity, there was a sense of freedom for me. He was always willing to do whatever I wanted and go wherever I wanted.

One day, he sat in his lounge chair in the living room, his lips pressed tight, his eyebrows knitted in a frown.

"Perry, are you okay?" I asked. "You look like you are frowning."

"I'm okay," he said, smiling.

"Are we treating you okay? Are we taking good care of you?"

"Yes," he said.

"What would you do if we weren't treating you okay or if we did something you didn't like? How would we know because you don't talk to us?"

He looked at me in surprise. "I would tell you to stop," he said.

I considered his response, pleasantly surprised. He was right, he did let his needs be known, like the day I pulled into the parking lot at a grocery store and he said, "No, I don't feel like grocery shopping," then refused to get out of the car. Or the time at a restaurant, when I tried to pull him in to the empty ladies room to change his diaper and he dug in his heels and stopped walking because he didn't want to go in the women's restroom. But most of the times, he went along with my choices or would say to me, "You decide," when I asked him what he preferred.

It was now entirely up to me to plan our days, our vacations, our activities and, I realized, I could do whatever I wanted. In the past, the simple act of seeing a movie would turn into a contest of wills. Perry loved violent, shoot-them-up movies while I preferred comedies and foreign films. There would be a period of compromise and trade-offs, we would see his movie this time but next time it would be my turn. Now, it was always my turn and I could determine our path.

I turned back to Ellen across the dinner table and smiled. "I don't know if fun is the word but I go on walks at the marina with Perry. We go to the Farmer's Market on Saturday. I'm into cooking again and we have dinner with our neighbors, Manny and Nancy, every Friday." I picked up my glass of wine and took a sip. "I appreciate small joys like reading a book and lying on the couch watching TV."

This was the shape of my life now.

CHAPTER 41

～╲╱～

On a lazy Saturday afternoon at home, I sat on the couch going through mail and browsing catalogues. When I saw the suede jacket in the Territory Ahead catalogue, I paused and caught my breath. I could imagine the pre-brain injury Perry in the bomber style jacket pictured on the page. The light brown suede, buttery and soft, would fit his coloring perfectly. A wave of longing for the old Perry washed over me like a hot flash, moving through my entire body from the small of my back to the tips of my toes. Even my gums ached with wistfulness for what used to be, what could have been.

I leaned my head back on the couch and closed my eyes. Glimpses of our old life appeared, bicycle rides along the beach from Playa del Rey to Hermosa Beach, long walks in the neighborhood through Sunset Park and Penmar Park, hikes in the Sierras and local Santa Monica mountains. I could hear Perry telling me the same joke, "*Is your nose running? Do your feet smell? You must be upside down!*" and me laughing. I pictured the dozen long stemmed red roses that would appear on my birthday and our anniversary or the jewelry, diamond earrings or pearls, he gave me at Christmas.

I imagined what our lives would have been without his brain injury. We could have commuted downtown together, both of us working late into the evening, calling to see if we were ready to make the drive home. Or maybe we would have met at one of the new restaurants downtown for cocktails and dinner since we no longer had children waiting at home, no dog to feed and no reason to be home at a certain hour.

We would have traveled together to all those exotic locations we had dreamed about: Paris, Rome, Istanbul or maybe returned to London. I would have gone with him to Christmas Island or the Cook Islands to satisfy his fishing desires. We would have resumed our annual backpacking trips into the Sierras, gone snowshoeing in Yellowstone, visited the Northern Lights and the lightning field in New Mexico.

Would we have remodeled the house or moved to a larger home? He would have taken his boat out every weekend when we lived in the marina during the remodel. We would have gone for walks arm in arm, instead of me pushing him in a wheelchair along the channels of the marina. We would have unpacked in the newly remodeled house together, him fussing with the speakers and wiring. He would have been the point of contact for the contractor and would have known how to install the light bulbs on the cylindrical light fixtures on the patio or make the Blue Ray player work.

I opened my eyes. The Saturday afternoon light was fading and the wind had picked up, rustling the leaves of the camphor tree on the street. A plane droned in the background at the Santa Monica airport but the street was quiet. My life was now defined by the confines of disability but for a few brief moments, it felt glorious to dream about what could have been and take comfort in all that was.

How was I to know that it would all be over so soon, that the life we once had would end on that fateful day on June 6, 2003? That day, at the airport lounge, he had tucked a bag of Fritos and an apple in my purse as we were leaving to board the plane.

"For later," he had said, with a smile. But how were we to know there would be no "later"?

Since that night in Portland, I have debated in my mind over and over whether it would have been better if he had just passed away and not been resuscitated. And there have been countless days in the throes of caregiving when life seemed unbearable and I wished that his body would just give out, that he would release us from the misery of brain injury.

And yet life without him seemed equally unbearable. There were the moments when I caught sight of his rounded forehead or the nape of his neck and I felt that same fluttering in my heart as I did in college. I had fallen in love with the Perry that emerged. I was comforted by his presence, even though he didn't speak much. I loved how he sang along with the Beatles when we drove in the car, how he always patted me on the butt whenever I reached down to help him with his shoes, how he mumbled in his sleep. I loved the way his sigh caught in his throat as he drifted off to sleep and his soft snores in the middle of the night. I loved his scent as he held me close to his chest, the way he puckered his lips for a kiss whenever I put my face close to his. I loved the way his eyes sparkled when he saw me and how he always answered, "Whatever you want to do," when asked how he wanted to spend the day. Enough of his essence remained so that his silent companionship anchored me, provided me with reminders of what was most important in life.

Besides, this slowed down life was not so bad. I thought of the walks we took along the bike path in Playa del Rey, the sun warming our backs, the glistening water from the canals. We had traveled the world to find that same sense of serenity but it was here, in our own backyard. Our circle of friends had dwindled but I was content with the pace of our lives. It was restful and peaceful. I had changed and grown since his brain injury. The world did not end for me when Perry gasped and stopped breathing. We had carved a new pathway.

I closed the catalogue on my lap and placed it on the coffee table. I got up from the couch and stepped toward Perry, who was sitting in his recliner chair, eyes closed, his head nodding from side to side. I tapped his hand and he opened his eyes. His face melted into a smile, his eyes wide and alert when he saw me.

"I have some work to do in the den," I said. "Do you want to come in the den with me or stay in the living room and watch TV?"

He smiled back at me.

"Go in the den with you," he said. "I want to be wherever you are."

On April 30, 2018, Perry passed away with Zack, Paul, his sister Amy and me by his side. There are no words to describe the emptiness of losing him and not being able to squeeze his hand, kiss his cheek, brush his forehead, see his smile or the light in his eyes.

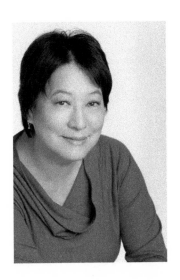

Cynthia Lim lives in Los Angeles. She is retired from the Los Angeles Unified School District and holds a doctorate in social welfare. Her essays have appeared in various publications including *Hawai'i Pacific Review*, *Gemini Magazine*, *Hobart*, and *Witness Magazine*. Find out more about Cynthia at www.cynthialimwriting.com.

CPSIA information can be obtained
at www.ICGtesting.com
Printed in the USA
FSHW01n2322061018
52770FS